Aging, Spirituality and Palliative Care

Aging, Spirituality and Palliative Care has been co-published simultaneously as *Journal of Religion, Spirituality & Aging,* Volume 18, Numbers 2/3 and 4 2006.

Aging, Spirituality and Palliative Care

Elizabeth MacKinlay, PhD, RN
Editor

Aging, Spirituality and Palliative Care has been co-published simultaneously as *Journal of Religion, Spirituality & Aging*, Volume 18, Numbers 2/3 and 4 2006.

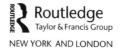

Routledge
Taylor & Francis Group

NEW YORK AND LONDON

First Published by

The Haworth Pastoral Press®, 10 Alice Street, Binghamton, NY 13904-1580 USA

Transferred to Digital Printing 2011 by Routledge
711 Third Ave, New York NY 10017
2 Park Square, Milton Park, Abingdon, Oxon, OX14 4RN

Aging, Spirituality and Palliative Care has been co-published simultaneously as *Journal of Religion, Spirituality and Aging*™, Volume 18, Numbers 2/3 and 4 2006.

Cover design by Kerry E. Mack

Library of Congress Cataloging-in-Publication Data

Aging, spirituality and palliative care /Elizabeth MacKinlay, editor.
  p. cm.
  Based on presentations made at the at The Third International Conference on Ageing and Spirirtuality held in Adelaide in 2004.
  "Co-published simultaneously as Journal of religion, spirituality & aging, volume 18, numbers 2/3 and 4 2006."
  Includes bibliographical references and index.
  ISBN-13: 978-0-7890-3341-3 (hard cover : alk. paper)
  ISBN-10: 0-7890-3341-0 (hard cover : alk. paper)
  ISBN-13: 978-0-7890-3342-0 (soft cover : alk. paper)
  ISBN-10: 0-7890-3342-9 (soft cover : alk. paper)
  1. Older people–Care–Congresses 2. Older people–Medical care–Congresses. 3. Older people–Religious life–Congresses . 4. Palliative treatment–Congresses 5. Death–Congresses. 6. Spirituality–Congresses I. MacKinlay, Elizabeth, 1940- II. International Conference on Ageing, Spirituality, and Palliative Care (2004 : Adelaide, S. Aust.) III. Journal of religion, spirituality & aging.
 HV1451.A45 2006
 362.198′97–dc22   2006002551

Aging, Spirituality and Palliative Care

CONTENTS

ABOUT THE EDITOR

Elizabeth MacKinlay, PhD, RN, is a registered nurse and an ordained priest in the Anglican Church of Australia, Associate Professor in the School of Theology at Charles Sturt University, and Director for the Centre for Ageing and Pastoral Studies. In addition, she is a member of the Anglican Retirement Community Services Board of Management for the diocese of Canberra and Goulburn. Dr. MacKinlay is a co-editor of *Aging, Spirituality, and Pastoral Care: A Multinational Perspective,* and editor of *Mental Health and Spirituality in Later Life,* and *Spirituality of Later Life: On Humor and Despair* (all from Haworth). Currently she is Principal Researcher in the research center of the Public and Contextual Theology (PACT) at Charles Sturt University.

Foreword

Palliative care in modern society offers a rich new frontier where things that are old are new and those that are new are often actually quite old. Care for persons with chronic illness and/or who are dying has taken place since the beginning of time. For thousands of years, spiritual caregivers were the only persons who were available for support. Yet, in more recent times, medicine and science have taken over this process, shifting the emphasis to physical comfort away from religious and spiritual care. Advances in medicine are important in their contributions to the quality of life in these times. However, emotional and spiritual care is still needed.

For chaplains in hospitals, one of the very clear roles is at the time of death. In the emergency room, the chaplain offers comfort to families and to patients, but they also need to stay out of the way of medical teams as they do their work to preserve life. However, if the person dies, then the chaplain is generally in charge of the intervention, not the physician. Once a patient has died, the chaplain's role becomes clearly to offer comfort to the family and to support decision-making in terms of funeral homes and the disposition of the body. Indeed at times the chaplain is the guardian of the body to be sure that it is treated respectfully and in concert with the belief system of the patient and their family. When possible, chaplains prefer to be a presence to both patient and family in advance of a death; however, this is the role of palliative care, not the emergency room.

Hospice care is another element of palliative care. Designed to be in-patient as with so many of the new medical innovations of the 1960s and 1970s and yet today it has become more of a home-based intervention. For chaplains, nurses and other spiritual caregivers, hospice offers a unique format to be able to listen to the patient and their family, understand their beliefs and spiritual needs, and then to offer support as

[Haworth co-indexing entry note]: "Foreword." Ellor, James W. Co-published simultaneously in *Journal of Religion, Spirituality & Aging* (The Haworth Pastoral Press, an imprint of The Haworth Press, Inc.) Vol. 18, No. 2/3, 2006, pp. xxv-xxvi; and: *Aging, Spirituality and Palliative Care* (ed: Elizabeth MacKinlay) The Haworth Pastoral Press, an imprint of The Haworth Press, Inc., 2006, pp. xv-xvi. Single or multiple copies of this article are available for a fee from The Haworth Document Delivery Service [1-800-HAWORTH, 9:00 a.m. - 5:00 p.m. (EST). E-mail address: docdelivery@haworthpress.com].

needed. Hospice, while relatively new, brings the patient back to focus on the dying process and comfort, rather than the more medically driven acute care models.

Life should not be reduced to the significance of the list days, yet in the last days we often tell the story of a life lived. When queried about death, older adults talk about a fear of how they will die, not in death itself. Older adults no longer experience the kind of death that is dramatically shown in the media where one knows that she or he is dying and turns to a trusted friend to say something profound, before gasping one last time and dying. Modern healthcare has altered these stereotypes, rendering most seniors helpless and speechless in the dying process. Too often chronic illness and the dying process is experienced alone. Not because families have abandoned them, but because the transition to medical care can inhibit the kind of surrounded family care that is closer to the memorialized ideal from years gone by. Whether in an institution or at home, whether the patient is able to speak for her or himself or not, spiritual care clearly involves getting in touch with the story of the person and finding the meaning of a life lived.

Spiritual care is not new. It is as old as the religions themselves. In early times it provided the majority of the care given to persons at times of chronic illness or who are dying. While at times it seems like modern society has strayed away from spiritual care at times of death, chaplains, hospice staff and volunteers, and numerous other key caregivers are still there surrounding the individual and family as appropriate. Spiritual care has moved from being the primary caregiver, to being a member of a team. Yet, whenever possible the individual is still surrounded by those who care and can work toward supportive care. In the pages of this volume, the stories of this team and the many voices that can be heard working together can be heard. It is an important topic that reflects both that which is old and yet that which is still new and in many ways under-addressed in the current literature.

James W. Ellor, PhD, DMin, DCSW

Preface

There are both opportunities and challenges as we face our own ageing and the ageing of societies. How people care for the older members
of their society tells much of the values held by that society. Care and
compassion, and respect for the weak and vulnerable of a society are
important measures of the physical and moral well being of that society.

In many parts of the world advances in public health, medicine and
technology have led to increased levels of health in later life; the positive ageing movement spells out the need for physical health for a better
quality of life in ageing. But there is yet more.

If life is to be worth living, there must also be meaning in that life.
The fulfillment of longer life cannot be just added years, but also the
need to find meaning in those years. The burden of chronic illness and
suffering still challenge us. But there is something more, the spark of
life, the yearning of the human spirit, of the soul. For humans have the
capacity to hope and to transcend the most difficult of times and experiences, the capacity to thrive and flourish. It is of the spiritual dimension
of ageing that this publication is concerned.

This collection of papers is based on presentations made at the Third
International Conference on Ageing and Spirituality. The first conference on ageing and spirituality took the focus of ageing, spirituality, and
pastoral care, the second, ageing, spirituality, and well-being; this third
conference includes a perspective on palliative care. Western societies
largely deny ageing and death and this book seeks to bring themes of
ageing, spirituality, and palliative care together to intentionally reclaim
the final career of life. This seems timely; in an ageing society with low
levels of mortality in early life, few people experience death first hand
until much later in life. Research shows that many older people do not
fear death, but do fear the process of dying. It is a journey that is new to
each one of us, as we come to our own final career–the process of dying.

[Haworth co-indexing entry note]: "Preface." MacKinlay, Elizabeth. Co-published simultaneously in
Journal of Religion, Spirituality & Aging (The Haworth Pastoral Press, an imprint of The Haworth Press, Inc.)
Vol. 18, No. 2/3, 2006, pp. xxvii-xxix; and: *Aging, Spirituality and Palliative Care* (ed: Elizabeth MacKinlay)
The Haworth Pastoral Press, an imprint of The Haworth Press, Inc., 2006, pp. xvii-xix. Single or multiple cop-
ies of this article are available for a fee from The Haworth Document Delivery Service [1-800-HAWORTH,
9:00 a.m. - 5:00 p.m. (EST). E-mail address: docdelivery@haworthpress.com].

It is a career that we would want to make well, for ourselves and for our loved ones.

The aims of this conference were to, first, explore the growing knowledge and practice base of ageing and spirituality; second, bring researchers and practitioners together to examine spirituality in later life, ways of growing spiritually in later life and strategies for providing best practice in aged care. The final aim of the conference was to examine the latest developments in palliative care and ageing.

Part I of the book begins with articles that reflect the state of the art in ageing and spirituality. First, Harriet Mowat's paper explores Scottish health care and the spiritual imperative. Dr. Mowat alerts us to three possible discourses of ageing: first, a problem to be solved, second, or the counter argument that ageing is not a problem, and third, ageing is a spiritual exploration. Robert Atchley's paper addresses aspects of continuity theory and spiritual development, with threads and spirals of continuity within a framework of reference points that constantly evolve throughout life.

Bruce Rumbold's paper considers the spirituality of compassion, touching on the importance of relationship and community. Rosalie Hudson explores spirituality as fragmentation, asking questions of the concept of person as an 'ensouled body' and 'embodied soul.' Issues of definition of spirituality emerged in a number of papers, and spiritual assessment was the topic of the paper by Elizabeth MacKinlay. John Killick shares wonderful images of people living with dementia, highlighted in the poem of the dying candle, where the flame burns just as brightly, even when much of the candle has already burned.

The article by Corinne Trevitt and Elizabeth MacKinlay reports findings of a study of spiritual reminiscence work with frail older people with dementia. Paul Winks' article examines fear of death, religiousness, and spirituality in later life. Michael Barbato's paper focused on the pain of dying, and how we mostly experience death as outsiders, unless it is the death of someone very close to us. David Currow and Meg Hegarty address concepts of suffering in palliative care, while both sorrow and joy are explored in the paper by Jenny Thompson-Richards (Dr. Wooops) on being a clown doctor.

The conference was attended by people from a number of religious and faith perspectives. Increasingly, Western countries are becoming multicultural and multifaith societies. As we discover more on this journey of ageing, we are mindful both of our Christian roots, but also of the presence of other faith and cultural traditions among us. In an ageing society it is important that our elders are able to practice their faith in freedom according to their beliefs and practices. Thus those of us who work with older people must be sensitive to the variety of need. The paper by Ruwan Palapathwala explores Buddhist and Christian perspectives on dying. The importance of relationship with others and love as agape in dying patients is emphasized in Ann Harrington's paper.

All people should have the opportunity to share their final journey with others. In a death denying society this final career needs to be reclaimed. Perhaps a midwife is needed to walk with those who are dying. Part II of this publication focuses on providing appropriate care for older people who are dying, with important papers by Linda Kristjanson, Laurie Grealish, and Margaret O'Connor and Susan Lee. These papers challenge the reader to look at experiences of dying, to change practices, consider ways of learning to provide appropriate care to older adults.

I wish to acknowledge and thank Karen Woodward for her valuable assistance in editing, and Graham Lindsay for his work on the figures.

Elizabeth MacKinlay, PhD, RN

PART I

Ageing Health Care
and the Spiritual Imperative:
A View from Scotland

Harriet Mowat, PhD

SUMMARY. This paper, given as a keynote presentation at the third international conference on Ageing and Spirituality 2004 in Adelaide, Australia, offers a perspective on ageing that makes central and fundamental the spiritual journey. Ageing is not confined to the old. We are all ageing all the time and whilst the imperative of ego integration (Erikson, 1986, 1982) is more pressing in old age, the march of time makes no exceptions. The paper starts with a consideration of the Scottish context and the current interest in Scotland in spirituality and health. Borrowing from the human developmental ideas of Frankl, Jung, Erikson, and Klein, the paper takes the view that we are all spiritual beings, and we are all trying to be successful, integrated reconciled and mature individuals. Ageing and spirituality is relevant to every individual. Successful ageing

Harriet Mowat, PhD, is Managing Director, Mowat Research, Ltd., 23 Carden Place, Aberdeen, AB10 1UQ, Scotland. She also is Professor, Robert Gordon University, Faculty of Health and Social Care, Aberdeen; Senior Research Associate, Queen Margaret University College, Centre for the Older Person's Agenda; Senior Research Fellow, University of Paisley School of Nursing and Midwifery; Senior Lecturer, Aberdeen University, Centre for Rural Studies; and Senior Lecturer, Aberdeen University, Centre for the Study of Spirituality, Disability, and Health.

[Haworth co-indexing entry note]: "Ageing Health Care and the Spiritual Imperative: A View from Scotland." Mowat, Harriet. Co-published simultaneously in *Journal of Religion, Spirituality & Aging* (The Haworth Pastoral Press, an imprint of The Haworth Press, Inc.) Vol. 18, No. 2/3 , 2006, pp. 3-17; and: *Aging, Spirituality and Palliative Care* (ed: Elizabeth MacKinlay) The Haworth Pastoral Press, an imprint of The Haworth Press, Inc., 2006, pp. 3-17. Single or multiple copies of this article are available for a fee from The Haworth Document Delivery Service [1-800-HAWORTH, 9:00 a.m. - 5:00 p.m. (EST). E-mail address: docdelivery@haworthpress.com].

Available online at http://www.haworthpress.com/web/JRSA
© 2006 by The Haworth Press, Inc. All rights reserved.
doi:10.1300/J078v18n02_01

is fundamentally concerned with the successful self. The spiritual journey is bound up with the search for meaning. Ageing is part of the task of being human and it involves decline and loss. The spiritual journey–search for meaning–is unique to each one of us. The spiritual journey is made evident in the search for the ultimate destination of giving up self, transcending self. Remembrance and routine are methods by which the ageing and the spiritual journey can be facilitated. A successful ageing, according to this perspective, is therefore one that embraces and self-consciously embarks upon a spiritual journey. To take it further–the spiritual journey is bound up with ageing–and further still–ageing is a spiritual journey (Bianchi, 1984). The primary task of ageing is spiritual development. Spiritual development is helped by an appropriate societal context in which ageing as spiritual journey can flourish. This has implications for health and social care services. *[Article copies available for a fee from The Haworth Document Delivery Service: 1-800-HAWORTH. E-mail address: <docdelivery@haworthpress.com> Website: <http://www.HaworthPress.com> © 2006 by The Haworth Press, Inc. All rights reserved.]*

KEYWORDS. Ageing, Scotland, older people, spiritual journey, spiritual need, caring task

SCOTLAND'S CHANGING SPIRITUAL LANDSCAPE

Increasing Interest in Spirituality and Health

An examination of the spiritual landscape in Scotland throws up some interesting observations. In line with much of Western Europe there is a significant decrease in adherence to traditional, formal institutional religion (Davie, 1994). The decreasing number of people regularly attending places of worship evidences this (Scottish Census, 2002). However, whilst traditional religion appears to be in decline, there is a corresponding *increase* in the number of people expressing the importance of spirituality for their lives and claiming to have spiritual experiences and beliefs (Hay, 1990). Spirituality appears to have migrated from the overtly religious towards a more individualistic and subjective quest that has no necessity of a formal structure, doctrinal beliefs or an anchoring community of like-minded believers (Heelas et al., 2005). People now want to *believe* in things spiritual, but no longer wish to *belong* to traditional religious institutions (Davie, 1994).

This broadening understanding of spirituality is reflected in health care settings by the increasing focus on spirituality within the literature surrounding medicine, nursing, social work, and occupational therapy,[1] a rising interest in complementary and alternative medicine (Austin, 1998), and a developing holistic view of health and illness within which the role of chaplaincy is rapidly gaining recognition.

Expanding Spirituality from the Particular to the Universal

In an environment that highly values the role of the "specialist," such a holistic view of health presents very particular challenges to individual professions and to the ways in which multi-disciplinary teams function in practice. As medicine and health care advance in knowledge of the micro mechanisms of the ill body, so the need for greater specialisation increases. In tension with this emphasis is the practical need expressed by people encountering illness to be treated as whole persons who require the universal (overarching meaning) and the particular (the individual self) to be held in critical tension throughout their experience of illness. Within such a context spirituality becomes of foremost importance.

In order to provide authentic holistic, active, total care, attention should be given to providing appropriate services that meet the *actual* needs of patients and their carers, that is, not simply the needs that health care professionals may perceive or/and assume, without reference to the wishes, desires and experiences of patients. The concept of patient focussed care is currently central to Scottish/UK Government health care policy, which stresses the importance of patient and carer views informing service developments. There is a good deal of evidence that suggests that patients desire to have their spiritual needs met within a healthcare context (Murray et al., 2004). Developing strategies to meet such expressed needs is therefore very much part of current governmental approach. Spirituality and spiritual care are not optional extras for "religious people."

Religion and Health–The Known Research

In the light of these cultural changes it is not coincidental that spirituality and religion are fast becoming recognised as a significant part of the healthcare research agenda, even amongst those more inclined towards the biomedical end of the research community spectrum (Fry, 2000). The extensive research work of people such as Harold Koenig and David Larson in the United States is indicative of the possibility of developing an evidence base to explore the possibility of there being a positive association between religion, spirituality and health (Larson et al., 1997; Koenig, 2001).

A similar evidence base to that being produced within the United States has still to be developed within the United Kingdom and Europe. It is therefore not possible to draw direct comparisons across cultures. Nevertheless, the evidence that does exist is helpful in locating some potential benefits spirituality and religion could offer at a clinical as well as a pastoral level.

THE POLICY CONTEXT IN SCOTLAND

Patient Focus and Public Involvement

In Scotland, the current and previous Ministers of Health have promoted the philosophy of patient focused care. Patient Focus and Public Involvement[2] (PFPI) was launched in December 2001 following key commitments within Designed to Care[3] and Our National Health: A plan for action, a plan for change.[4] The Partnership Agreement[5] commits the Scottish Executive to addressing the following themes in all its work:

- Growing Scotland's economy;
- Delivering excellent public services;
- Supporting stronger, safer communities; and
- Developing a confident, democratic Scotland.

In line with these themes, National Health Service (NHS) Scotland is committed to equality, excellence, and the provision of high quality health services across Scotland. The leadership for this commitment comes from both the Minister for Health and Community Care and the Chief Executive of NHS Scotland.

Key to the provision of this culture of continuous improvement in clinical quality is the involvement of patients, services users, their families and the public in the design, development and delivery of the services they use. The health plan outlined in the document "Our National Health: a plan for action, a plan for change" therefore committed NHS Scotland to giving patients a stronger voice and involving people and communities in the design and delivery of health services.

PFPI developed the Health Plan commitments into a framework for change that covered the entire breadth and depth of NHS Scotland.

The White Paper, Partnership for Care[6] set out a vision of a patient-focused National Health Service based on a new partnership between patients and staff. Meeting the challenge of Partnership for Care means ensuring that whatever the individual circumstances of someone's life, they have access to the right health services to meet their needs. This includes their spiritual needs.

The NHS Reform (Scotland) Act 2004 now underpins these Partnership for Care commitments and places specific duties on NHS Boards to involve the public and promote equality of opportunity. The Act also provides for the establishment of a Scottish Health Council, with a distinctive identity within NHS Quality Improvement Scotland. These bodies will quality assure NHS Boards' delivery of their patient focus and public involvement commitments on behalf of the people of Scotland.

In relation to spiritual care there is clearly a need for some understanding of spirituality among all health service staff. The focus over the last three years (2000-2004) has been on understanding and supporting the development of spiritual care policies in every Health Board area in Scotland. Scottish Health Care Chaplaincy has been identified as the obvious location for a new kind of spiritual care which appeals to all faiths and none. There are challenges in moving from a largely Church of Scotland based chaplaincy service to one that represents and supports people from all faiths and none (Mowat and Swinton, 2005).

Spiritual Care Guidelines

At the same time and in response to the types of changes and developments highlighted earlier, a steering group was set up to explore what was required in terms of enabling chaplains to provide effective spiritual care. This group produced a set of guidelines for good practice. This process resulted in a Health Department Letter (HDL) to all Health Boards providing guidance on the development of local policies, which are being steered and developed by hospital chaplains and other staff; two conferences aimed at senior Trust management; and the setting up of a Chaplaincy Training and Development and Spiritual Care Coordinating Unit. Each Board is developing local spiritual care policies and these are being implemented by the chaplains, lead managers, and widely representative Spiritual Care committees.

Spirited Scotland

The Scottish Executive Health Department has funded an initiative known as *Spirited Scotland*, which offers a broad perspective on Spirituality and Health in Scotland (Mowat and Ryan, 2003). It acts as a networking point, hosts a website and issues a newsletter. In practical terms it has supported the development of confidence amongst health and social care staff to deal with spiritual issues by offering educational initiatives within the Trusts. A newly formed *Centre for Spirituality, Health and Disability*, at the University of Aberdeen,[7] is also pursuing a research and development agenda that promises to make a significant contribution to the area of spirituality and health care.

It is clear then that, within Scotland, there is an important movement to take healthcare in directions which meet the types of spiritual need prevalent within contemporary culture.

The largest proportion of patients in the NHS is over 65. This group of older people have particular challenges. They are likely to experience multiple pathology, age-related vicissitudes, and anxieties about their own ageing and mortality. The spiritual imperatives experienced by these people are likely to affect their well-being and experience of ageing.

AGEING AND THE SEARCH FOR MEANING

Ageing is part of the task of being human. It involves decline and loss. The spiritual journey is bound up with the search for meaning. To paraphrase T.S. Eliot, an English 20th Century poet, there are two fundamental questions in life. Firstly, what does life mean and secondly, what are we going to do about it? Both as individuals, and as a society, our various discourses concerning ageing are a more or less helpful means of handling such questions. I will argue below that the search for meaning in ageing is fundamentally a spiritual task, unique to each one of us, yet common to all. It is what binds us together and also what prompts us to isolate ourselves from each other. A discourse which acknowledges this can assist both the older person and the carer to create or locate meaning in the aging process (Seeber, 1990). A successful ageing according to this perspective, is therefore one that embraces and self consciously embarks upon a spiritual journey (Mowat, 2003). To take it further–the spiritual journey is bound up with ageing–and further still–ageing is a spiritual journey.

AGEING AND THE INDIVIDUAL–BALANCING DISCOURSES

In order to give substance to the idea of the various discourses that can be in operation simultaneously we will briefly consider the different situations of Pam and Angus.

Pam, aged 54, complained of stomach pain. Within one week of consulting the General Practitioner about her symptoms she was given a diagnosis of pancreatic cancer with liver secondaries. Her dilemma became how to continue living with that knowledge. What could be her *method* of daily life in a world that held no promise of tomorrow?

Her method became apparent. She held in her mind two ways of viewing her situation: two assumptions or discourses. Firstly, she made an assumption of immortality. She would recover despite the odds of recovery and she embraced vigorously plans for her future. Secondly, she made an assumption of mortality. She spoke clearly about her imminent death. She acknowledged the importance of living in the moment without reference to the future.

She operated these personal discourses concurrently. Sometimes they appeared within the same sentence. Her visitors became aware that she required them to keep up with these discourses and respond appropriately. Her visitors had the role of offering her confirmation of both these assumptions. These two assumptions were both of extreme importance to Pam in her struggle to come to terms with her situation.

Angus is 84. He is married to Sheila who is 69. They married two years ago, two years after Angus' first wife Mary died. Sheila is an old family friend. Angus is very happy indeed with Sheila and sees himself as fortunate to have met two women with whom he could live in great harmony in his lifetime.

Angus has a number of symptoms and visits the general practitioner regularly–he is highly motivated to remain healthy and well, given his relatively new marital status. He views himself as a naturally cheerful individual. Most of his contemporaries and long-term friends from college days are either dead or have cancer. A weekly phone call to his daughter includes a catalogue of funerals, terminal illnesses and disabling conditions belonging to others.

Angus, like Pam, also operates two discourses, but he only *engages* with one–the assumption of immortality. Angus acts as though his life span will continue indefinitely. He rarely discusses the possibility of his own demise despite his age and he plans ahead for holidays and events years hence.

Angus was unable to speak with his first wife about her impending death. He has not allowed himself to be confronted with a situation that has made him face, in stark terms, his own mortality, his own ageing. He looks well and young for his age. He still plays golf–his aches and pains are related to age rather than illness. Angus' two discourses are not balanced. This potentially leaves him very vulnerable if his lifestyle and life circumstances are radically changed through ill health.

MAINTENANCE OF BALANCE

As we progress through life, our life voices are a balance between immortality and imminence. We must have both these discourses to progress–but they move in and out of focus depending on our current circumstances. Ageing is a process of maintaining a balance in the discourses of immortality and imminence so that we can manage ourselves and our lives and maximise our meaning.

Our carers and helpers, our family and friends must learn to follow our balance which changes on a daily basis–this involves careful listening and observing, the real work of compassionate caring. Pam's story shows that listeners to the discourse must also learn to move with the emphasis between immortality and imminence that prevails at any one moment.

AGEING AND SOCIETY–TWO DISCOURSES

Scottish society also seems to work with two ageing discourses. At first glance they are very different. In what could be called the *problem based discourse*, ageing is assumed to be difficult and essentially a problem both for the individual and society. Conversely, ageing is portrayed as the advent of wisdom and an opportunity for both the individual and society.

Both these discourses have implications for the individual and the perception of successful ageing. Both these discourses seem to share the same underpinning assumptions although they look somewhat different superficially.

FIRST DISCOURSE:
THE PROBLEM BASED THEORY OF AGEING

In our current Scottish society, ageing is most commonly seen as something to be feared and rejected. Ageing is something to be ignored.

Ageing is something that happens to other people. Ageing is a problem to "fix" through social, economic, or health policy. Ageing is a biological "mistake" or challenge that will eventually be rectified through scientific endeavour (Kirkwood, 2000).

The problem based discourse around ageing can be understood as a fear of death and the instinctual drive towards denial of death. In a secular environment the reality of death has the potential to render life meaningless. Meaning of life questions, in our current society, are bound up with maintenance of youth and continuity of "youthful" practice. When illness occurs, as it does increasingly with old age, the individual is required, mostly unwillingly, to reflect on his or her position and the meaning of his/her life in a wider context.

This problem based approach to ageing could be considered to be similar to the psychological position known as the paranoid-schizoid, which is described by Kleinian psychotherapy (Greenberg and Mitchell, 1983). In this position the relationship to the object, in this case ageing and death, is very stark and uncompromising and places the perceiver in a difficult and rigid position. Ageing is seen as a mistake to be rectified in due course. The underpinning assumption is that ageing is a "bad" thing. We find ourselves surprised by old age rather than planning for it. This perception of ageing is rooted in the wish to avoid the realities of ageing and death. By denying it, ageing loses its power to make us afraid. This is most often displayed by the denial of old age in oneself, but the recognition of it in others. Escaping or cheating old age also has a market value.

The research around ageing in this discourse tends to focus on collective solutions using a positivistic methodology. In this position successful ageing is defined by the clever avoidance or overcoming of the vicissitudes of old age. The successful ager is the one who escapes old age. Rewards are for people who "do not look their age" or who are "marvelous for their age." Medicine helps with this by improving techniques, for instance, hip replacements, heart bypass surgery, plastic surgery, sophisticated biomedical interventions. Social science helps by redefining the concept of elderly in terms of retirement age or in terms of pension rights and financial bonuses.

Since ageing and death are inevitable, the strongly held internal belief that ageing does not happen to self, only others, hosts the potential for anomie (Douglas, 1967), that is, dislocation from the mainstream structures of society and societal beliefs as the individual does relentlessly age.

In this position, society tends to associate the "blame" for ageing with those who create a problem around ageing. Those people who are creating a problem (by requiring services, taking pensions, using resources) tend to be stigmatised by society where blame is an important mechanism of social control. If the societal norm is to treat ageing as a problem then there will be a stigma against the old and a consequent discrimination.

SECOND DISCOURSE:
AGEING IS NOT A PROBLEM,
IT IS TO BE WELCOMED

The alternative view is that ageing brings with it wisdom and calm and releases energy. Even the vicissitudes associated with old age are to be embraced. Tom Kitwood's idea of personhood (Kitwood, 1997) exemplifies this counter view of the ageing process. This view comes from a variety of sources and disciplines and tends to be reinforced by qualitative studies looking at the *individual* perspective on ageing. (Achenbaum, 2001; Frieden, 1993) In these studies and in a longitudinal study by the author (Mowat, 1999), it is shown that ageing is not a problem for the individual; it is society and groups that find ageing difficult.

As a collective view, however, this optimistic view of ageing can also be seen as a denial. Here ageing is reconstructed as opportunity and maximisation of the creative individual self. Whilst it is not a denial of age it denies the need to take age seriously as decline and ultimately death. The underpinning assumption is that ageing has social benefits and creative opportunities for the individual and society, and these benefits must be acknowledged and exploited. It is driven by a challenge to ageism and age prejudice. It sees ageing as something to be constructed by the individual. Ageing is a creative negotiation. There is a focus on the wisdom of old age–old age as a golden age, although this is challenged by authors such as Woodward (2003) as being incompatible with anger and fighting for rights and a position in society. This perspective may simply reflect the hopes of those now entering old age.

Research tends to focus on the lived experience of ageing using a social construction perspective (Berger, 1969). In this position successful ageing is to live one's life to the full and to overcome and transcend the vicissitudes of old age and reject the stereotypes of the problem based model. Social science and practical gerontology have promoted this idea strongly in Scotland. The Dementia Services Development Centre at Stirling University is an example of a campaigning, almost evangelical organisation that promotes anti-ageist care and encourages a positive view of even the most devastating of illnesses associated with old age.

This position is potentially uncompromising and holds danger of being prescriptive. Its very attempt to regain the individual in old age leaves it open to reject those individuals who do not fit the creative individual prototype. Thus it becomes another model that could be described in object relations terms as paranoid-schizoid–the other side of the same coin.

A THIRD DISCOURSE:
AGEING AS A SPIRITUAL JOURNEY

The spiritual journey based theory of ageing is a maturation from the paranoid-schizoid position of good versus bad. It could be called a depressive position. In maturational terms this is considered to be a more balanced position to take.

If this can be called the depressive position it means that the individual/society is realistic in their understanding of their position–that they will grow old and that they will die. This approach is characterised by a search for meaning of self in relation to the wider society and world. The underpinning assumption is that ageing is inevitable, as is death and that there is loss and pain in the process of growing older (Kimble, 2002). The perception of ageing is rooted in its purpose as a vehicle for spiritual journey. Ageing is an important part of the spiritual journey and offers opportunity for growth and discovery of self through suffering and loss, which can be helped by attention to the creative self. The successful ager in this position is the ageing self who can both negotiate and retain meaning through discovery of self and who can then transcend self.

Viktor Frankl (1984) offers us a vision of humanity that moves away from reductionism and biological drives. Both offer us the opportunity to see human beings as essentially spiritual. Frankl suggests that human beings are spiritual beings with an irreducible core. This is expressed in a spiritual unconscious. The spiritual unconscious allows the mind to relate to what is not yet understandable or known, whereas the conscious mind can only relate to what is or what has been. The essence of the spiritual being is self transcendence.

If we take Frankl's irreducible spiritual core as given, then the task for the individual, the ageing individual is to discover and negotiate individual meaning, even when confronted with what Frankl calls the tragic triad of pain, guilt, and death. The task of old age and its fundamental purpose is therefore to search for meaning through a search for spiritual self. This is what Jung called individuation, Antonovsky called a sense of coherence and Erikson called ego integrity. The search for and maintenance of self can take place through remembrance. The remembrance of self is part of the manifestation of "attitude" that Frankl speaks of.

The implications of this perspective for a societal view on ageing are that ageing is seen as something universal and a bond between individuals and groups, rather than divisive and strange. The fear of death and dying implied by ageing may well be present but the method of coping with fears is inclusion rather than exclusion.

Our societal task both as individuals and groups is therefore to support people in their remembrance and exploration of self, to help them maintain the balance in their personal discourses between imminence and immortality and within society in a suitably mature depressive position.

PAST, PRESENT, AND FUTURE SELVES:
THE STRUGGLE FOR INTEGRITY

There are three selves that preoccupy us simultaneously: the past self, the present self and the future self. As we grow older the balance between these three selves shifts and the past self takes on a significance and importance which helps us understand our present and future selves. Each of these selves is uniquely related to each other. This gives us our individuality and our unique life story. However, none of us can escape the ego integration work that Erik Erikson so carefully identifies as the work of old age. According to Erikson, achieving a sense of integrity means fully accepting oneself and coming to terms with death. Accepting responsibility for your life and being able to accept the past and achieve satisfaction with self is essential. The inability to do this results in a feeling of despair.

The future self requires contemplation of our own mortality. We are required to face up to our own death. Remembering our forthcoming death puts into sharp relief our past self and present self. Who are we, why are we and what is next? This may well be the first time that we have thought of these questions and time seems to be running out. The ageing moment comes upon us unawares and we are caught in a situation that we may not have prepared for, both as individuals and as a society. Like illness the ageing moment forces us to contemplate our purpose. This is the challenge for the ageing self.

A central role for the carer of older people who are struggling with this task is to help them with the struggle rather than to prevent them struggling in an effort to avoid pain.

CONCLUSIONS

Implications for Those Working with Older People

The fundamental role of those working with older people is thus to maintain and sustain the self in the very situations that compromise that self, so that individuals can be free to do their spiritual work if they so choose. Knowledge of the context in which the older self has lived and worked is crucial. The self is maintained and made relevant through remembering–acts of remembrance become key components of the caring work.

By supporting older people through this process we also support ourselves, whatever age we are. We must pay attention to our own spiritual self, however, in order that we can be supportive to others.

As well as knowing the context of the older person with whom we work, we must also encourage an attitude of meaning. Viktor Frankl teaches us something of taking on such an attitude. His research and thinking tells us that the human spirit is irreducible. We are first and foremost spiritual beings. Our human task is to search for and assume meaning. Meaning is not invented but discovered. We do this through realising creative and experiential values.

Peter Speck (2001) has suggested that there needs to be greater cooperation between gerontologists, pastoral caregivers, sociologists, and health care providers in collaboration with discussions within society, if we are to be able to change towards more positive attitudes to ageing. This article hopes to contribute to this discussion by suggesting practical ways of being carers, companions and active participants on the spiritual journey into old age.

NOTES

1. For example Jessica Kingsley Publishers multidisciplinary series on spirituality and healthcare.

2. Scottish Executive (2001). *www.scotland.gov.uk/library3/health/pfpi-00.asp*

3. Designed to Care, SEHD (1997). *http://www.scotland.gov.uk/library/documents1/care-00.htm*

4. Scottish Executive (2000). *http://www.scotland.gov.uk/library3/health/onh-00.asp*

5. Scottish Executive (2003). http://www.scotland.gov.uk/library5/government/pfbs00.asp
  6. Scottish Executive (2000). *http://www.scotland.gov.uk/library3/health/onh-00.asp*
  7. The creation of The Centre for Spirituality, Health and Disability (2003). *http://www. abdn.ac.uk/newsletter/issue_24/story10.shtml*

REFERENCES

Achenbaum, W. A. (2001). Aging in Grace: The spiritual journey of Henri Nouwen. *Journal of Aging & Identity*, 6, 4, 183-219.

Antonovsky, A. (1987). *Unravelling the mysteries of health: How people manage stress and stay well*. Philadelphia: Josey Bass Wiley.

Austin, J. A. (1998). Why patients use alternative medicine: Results of a national study. *Journal of the American Medical Association*, 19, 1548-53.

Berger, P. (1969). *The social reality of religion*. London: Faber.

Bianchi, E. (1984). *Ageing as a spiritual journey*. New York: Crossroad Publishing Co.

Davie, G. (1994). *Religion in Britain since 1945: Believing without belonging*. Oxford: Blackwell.

Douglas, J. (1967). *The social meanings of suicide*. Boston: Princetown University Press.

Erikson, E. H., Erikson, J. M., & Kivnick, H. Q. (1986). *Vital involvement in old age*. New York: Norton.

Erikson, E. H. (1982). *The life cycle completed*. New York: Norton.

Frankl, V. (1984). *Man's search for meaning: An introduction to logotherapy*. Toronto: Touchstone Books.

Frieden, B. (1993). *The Fountain of Age*. New York: Simon and Schuster.

Fry, P. S. (2000). Religious involvement, spirituality, and personal meaning for life: Existential predictors of psychological wellbeing in community-residing and institutional care elders. *Aging & Mental Health*, 4, 4, 375-387.

Greenberg, J., & Mitchell, S. (1983). *Object relations in psychoanalytic theory*. Boston: Harvard University Press.

Hay, D. (1990). *Religious experience today: Studying the facts*. London: Cassell.

Heelas, P., Woodhead, L., Seel, B., Tusting, K., & Szerszynoki, B. (2005). *The spiritual revolution: Why religion is giving way to spirituality*. Oxford: Blackwell.

Kimble, M. (2002). *Viktor Frankl's contribution to spirituality and aging*. New York: The Haworth Pastoral Press.

Kirkwood, T. (2000). *Time of our lives*. London: Orion Books Ltd.

Kitwood, T. (1997). *Dementia reconsidered: The person comes first*. London: Open University Press.

Koenig, H., McCullough, M., & Larson, D. (2001). *Handbook of religion and health*. Oxford: Oxford University Press.

Larson, D., Sawyers, J. P., & McCullough, M. (1997). *Scientific research on spirituality and health: A consensus report*. Washington, DC: National Institute for Healthcare Research.

Moberg, D. O. (2001). *Ageing and spirituality: Spiritual dimensions of aging theory, research, practice, and policy*. New York: The Haworth Pastoral Press.

Mowat, H. (1999). *Expert elders and successful ageing: A series of presentations*. Information available from author.

Mowat, H., & Swinton, J. (2005). *What do Chaplains do? The role of the Chaplain in meeting the spiritual needs of patients*. Centre for Spirituality, Health and Disability, Aberdeen University Report No. CSHD/MR001 ISBN 0-9549901-0-2.

Mowat, H. (2003). The spiritual journey and successful ageing. In A. Jewell (Ed.), *Ageing, spirituality and wellbeing*. London: Jessica Kingsley Press.

Mowat, H., & Ryan, D. (2003). Spiritual issues in health and social care: Practice into policy? In S. McFadden, M. Brennan, & J. Patrick (Eds.), *New directions in the study of late life religiousness and spirituality*. New York: The Haworth Pastoral Press.

Murray, S., Kendall, M., Boyd, K., Worth, A., & Benton, T. (2004). Exploring the spiritual needs of people dying of lung cancer or heart failure: A prospective qualitative interview study of patients and their carers. *Palliative Medicine*, 18, 39-45.

Scottish Church Census (2002). *http://www.scottishchristian.com/features/0305census 01.shtml*

Scottish Executive (2001). *Cancer in Scotland: Action for change*. Edinburgh: Scottish Executive.

Scottish Executive (2003). *A new public involvement structure for NHS Scotland patient focus and public involvement*. *www.scotland.gov.uk/library3/health/pfpi-00.asp*

Scottish Executive (2000). *Our national health: A plan for action, a plan for change*. *http://www.scotland.gov.uk/library3/health/onh-00.asp*

Scottish Executive (2003). *A partnership for a better Scotland: Partnership agreement*. *http://www.scotland.gov.uk/library5/government/pfbs-00.asp*

Scottish Office (1997). *Designed to care*. *http://www.scotland.gov.uk/library/documents1/care-00.htm*

Seeber, J. (Ed.) (1990). *Spiritual maturity in later life*. New York: The Haworth Press, Inc.

Speck, P. (2001). *Spirituality and well being in women over 45 years*. Oxford: Pennell Initiative for Women's Health.

Woodward, K. (2003). Against wisdom: The social politics of anger and aging. *Journal of Aging Studies*, 1, 55-67.

Continuity, Spiritual Growth, and Coping in Later Adulthood

Robert C. Atchley, PhD

SUMMARY. Continuity of values, lifestyles, and relationships combines with spiritual growth in later life to provide most people a sense of direction and adequate resources for coping with changes that occur with aging. Being able to recognize threads of continuity and to perceive benefit from one's inner life are significant predictors of being able to maintain life satisfaction in the face of negative aspects of aging. Data from a 20-year longitudinal study are used to provide details. *[Article copies available for a fee from The Haworth Document Delivery Service: 1-800-HAWORTH. E-mail address: <docdelivery@haworthpress.com> Website: <http://www.HaworthPress.com> ©2006 by The Haworth Press, Inc. All rights reserved.]*

KEYWORDS. Continuity, spiritual development, coping

Despite a social world that has a negative orientation toward things aging, most aging and older people have good health, high self-acceptance and self-esteem, a high degree of life satisfaction, a satisfying and meaningful lifestyle, and a long-standing convoy of social support. This

Robert C. Atchley, PhD, is Chair, Department of Gerontology, Naropa University, 2130 Arapahoe Avenue, Boulder, CO 80302-6697 USA.

[Haworth co-indexing entry note]: "Continuity, Spiritual Growth, and Coping in Later Adulthood." Atchley, Robert C. Co-published simultaneously in *Journal of Religion, Spirituality & Aging* (The Haworth Pastoral Press, an imprint of The Haworth Press, Inc.) Vol. 18, No. 2/3, 2006, pp. 19-29; and: *Aging, Spirituality and Palliative Care* (ed: Elizabeth MacKinlay) The Haworth Pastoral Press, an imprint of The Haworth Press, Inc., 2006, pp. 19-29. Single or multiple copies of this article are available for a fee from The Haworth Document Delivery Service [1-800-HAWORTH, 9:00 a.m. - 5:00 p.m. (EST). E-mail address: docdelivery@haworthpress.com].

Available online at http://www.haworthpress.com/web/JRSA
© 2006 by The Haworth Press, Inc. All rights reserved.
doi:10.1300/J078v18n02_02

happens because over decades of life experience, a large majority of adults have developed robust ideas about what they want out of life and how to get it. Most people don't just sit back and let life happen, they try to influence the directions it takes for them. They usually understand that they don't *control* life's direction, but they believe they can *influence* it. They have enduring values that serve as the basis for their life structure, day-to-day decision-making, and their vision of a desired future. They are also resilient; they have encountered enough surprises, contradictions, and paradoxes in life to know that they have to pay attention and cope when the situation demands it. What they have learned from life is a powerful resource for coping. Most have also discovered that coping is easier when done with the support of others.

Focus on the inner life, service to others, and deepening connection with the sacred are bright spots of growth and development for most elders. Many elders see these trends as fully available to them and as goals around which they can organize their lives. The sense of optimism and equanimity that comes from leading this sort of life is also a great resource for coping.

When we see elders for whom things have gone awry, we can look to their personal systems for clues concerning unwanted discontinuities, an inadequate sense of meaning, and a murky view of where they are headed.

Thus, the strong coping capacity most elders possess rests on an equanimity that comes from continuity of values, lifestyles, and relationships plus turning to spirituality as a frontier of individual development and community formation. Continuity provides a benchmark for organizing thoughts and action; spiritual development provides a spacious context and an expansive perspective, which can foster a sense of equanimity even in the face of adversity.

We will explore each of these topics in more detail. Data to support the various ideas presented come from my 20-year longitudinal study of aging and adaptation (Atchley, 1999) and from my research on spiritual development and service in later adulthood (Atchley, 2000, 2003, 2004, 2005).

CONTINUITY

Continuity is dynamic and evolutionary. Like continuity in a stage play, continuity here means a character evolving over a lifetime of action and learning and struggle and joy and heartbreak. The character remains recognizable in most cases, but evolution is also obvious. Continuity of values and beliefs, lifestyles, and relationships constitutes a solid base from which to greet changes in circumstances, both positive and negative.

Based on a longitudinal study that began with 1,300 people age 50 or older in 1975 and followed them for 20 years, I was able to look at internal continuity of ideas and external continuity of activities and relationships as they adapted to aging. Details of this study were published in Atchley (1999).

Most people develop a personal system that is a result of decades of learning through life experience. Some people don't learn much from life, but most do. Their personal system is a reflection of their values and their experiences trying to live by them. Values are some of the most enduring inner constructs we have. They fuel our aspirations and our fears.

By late middle age, most adults have developed self-confidence, a feeling that they can influence their own fate. In fact, only about one percent of the people in my longitudinal study had low self-confidence. Most also have a high degree of emotional resilience. Health is the factor most likely to affect both self-confidence and emotional resilience, but even people who have poor health and functional disability seldom have low self-confidence or lack emotional resilience.

"Being able to accept myself as I am" is a very prevalent personal goal and becomes moreso over time. This reflects a shift in orientation from self-esteem based on feedback from others to self-esteem based on an inner integration, which Erikson, Erikson, and Kivnick (1986) referred to as integrity. Other important self-referent values include being dependable and reliable and being self-reliant. People want to be someone who can be counted on and to stand on their own two feet. They want to be seen as a good person by others. The resilience of these values even in the face of substantial disability suggests that as long as people can see these values at work in their lives in some fashion, self-respect can be maintained. And this self-respect is rooted in realism, not idealism.

In later adulthood, people also value *social connections* with family and friends, with family having primacy for most people. More than 80 percent feel it is important to have at least one close, intimate relationship. Having a confidant is important for both men and women.

By late adulthood, values such as being prominent in the community or being accepted by influential people are *unimportant* for most people.

I found a high prevalence of continuity over time in values, with 80 percent showing evolution within a basic value framework over the 20-year period.

Lifestyles are constructed to produce life satisfaction and life experience tells us how we are doing with that. By later life, most people have settled into a lifestyle that reflects their values and that is very robust in terms of helping people adapt to change.

Over the 20 years of my longitudinal study, continuity of activities occurred most commonly for reading (83.5%), being with friends (75.4%), being with family (67.5%), attending church (66.9%), and gardening (56.6%). Note that most of these activities are ones that an individual can easily adapt to changes in health. In overall activity patterns, very few people took up new activity areas as they aged. Most adjusted their level of participation in activities with which they already had experience. When I looked at how people adapted to functional loses, most were able to maintain the same activity pattern at a lower level of participation. This allowed them to continue to get satisfaction from the same lifestyle despite functional limitations or changes in living arrangements.

Life experience is filled with paradoxes, contradictions, and ambiguities. Relationships, especially the convoy of social support, help us understand the nuances of life, grapple with decision-making under conditions of uncertainty, and receive comfort in times of trial.

SPIRITUAL DEVELOPMENT

Spiritual development supplies new perspectives and motives that provide a renewed sense of direction in later life. It is promoted by questions such as:

> Is this all there is? What does it all mean? How do I fit into the picture? What will happen to me when I die? How can I leave a legacy for future generations? How can I give back to a world that has nurtured me? Do I need to get even with a world that hasn't nurtured me?

These and many other questions fuel a spiritual journey that for most people becomes serious in midlife. This happens as parents begin to age and experience frailty, as family and cohorts begin to die in larger numbers. It can also result from having been successful and finding that success doesn't provide the meaning we have been led to expect.

At its heart, the spiritual journey is about becoming rooted in being, about nurturing and living in a connection with the sacred, however labeled. It is also about developing a perspective about life that transcends the purely self-centered. Non-personal consciousness combines with spiritual development to create a channel for the universal love that is compassion. Compassion is a prerequisite for meaningful service. It takes a lot of compassion to be with others' suffering.

> Within each I Am lies the great source of all being
> Light from within, that's our illumination
> To dwell in silent peace and stillness, that's our meditation
> To see the passing world with clearness and compassion
> And when we clearly see, we are drawn to be love and to serve.

(Adapted from *The Journey*, Atchley, 1996)

Many elders participate in small circles of friends who support one another on their life journeys, including their spiritual journeys. There are also groups that focus their attention specifically on the spiritual journey. Many religious communities have numerous small groups that serve this purpose. They may be called study groups, women's groups, men's groups, or issue groups, but many of them also serve the purpose of providing support to the group members as they grapple with life issues, including spiritual development.

Not everyone is lucky enough to be part of a spiritual community that fosters such groups. The Spiritual Eldering Institute was created to promote inner spiritual work and recovering the role of spiritual elder in the community. It offers educational programs and resource material, especially concerning how to form, facilitate, or convene small groups aimed at spiritual development and spiritually-centered service (Spiritual Eldering Institute, 2004). The website, www.ServingFromSpirit. com, has similar aims.

The point here is that spiritual development often occurs spontaneously and naturally, but because it is an enjoyable purpose we may also be attracted to a conscious spiritual journey, either alone, in the company of others, or both.

Spiritual development is in essence an increasing connection with the nonpersonal, sacred Self that lies within each human being, whether they are religious or not. Spiritual development leads people toward deeper spiritual experience, an expansive view of time and space, and the joy of service for its own sake. For those drawn to it, spiritual experience gradually accompanies more and more of life until most experiences are at least partly a spiritual experience.

Joy in the act of serving comes to be its own reward and doesn't depend on social acknowledgement, so it is available all the time. Spiritual development creates increasingly large space in consciousness and in that large nonpersonal space, it is possible to see the ups and downs of the world with something approaching compassion and equanimity.

Most elders continue to serve their families, but in new ways that tap into the wisdom that comes with learning from a lifetime of experience. For most people, the role of grandparent is a wonderful mix of caring and mentoring, without the heavy child-rearing responsibilities of parenthood. It is one of later life's greatest service opportunities, and in it, we serve not only our grandchildren, but our children as well.

Most elders gradually learn compassionate listening, which creates space for younger people to express their hopes and fears and often opens the door for mentoring, which is in many ways the social equivalent of being a midwife. The mentor doesn't determine the nature of the new being, just eases the birth.

Most elders are part of circles of friends who support one another by providing a safe context for learning and coping. Often, elders are also very much in touch with nature's need for us to serve it. Caring for plants, animals and the natural environment seems like a very important way to be rooted in the earth.

Years of being on a path of service leads to an understanding that every contact with every thing can be an opportunity for service, so we don't have to worry about opportunities. We may have long-term service commitments we are willing to make, but we also are awake to opportunities that spontaneously arise to be helpful. To know what is needed, we must clearly see, which is very much a spiritual practice. Clear seeing demands that we be able to stand outside our personal agendas, and spiritual development promotes this process.

The website, www.ServingFromSpirit.com, is an effort designed to provide resources for those who want to deepen their spiritual connection and to live a life of spiritually-centered service. When we are committed to service, we see opportunities everywhere and we don't have to be preoccupied with whether we have the "authority" or are "required" to serve.

COPING

In combination, continuity and spiritual development explain why a large proportion of elders adapt well to the ups and downs of aging. But let us look more closely at the dynamics of coping.

Continuity is an adaptation strategy. When people need to adapt, more than 90 percent first try solutions that have worked for them in the past, use self knowledge to make decisions, and lean toward activities that have proved satisfying in the past. Nearly 90 percent have a personal philosophy of life that is a consistent force in the decisions they make.

In terms of specific patterns, how people adapt is highly individualized. But we can make a few general statements. First, relationships are a vital element of adaptation for most people. When asked, "What enables you to cope? What keeps you going?" family and friends are mentioned first by most people. Having a positive attitude is a close second. This is expressed in many ways: sense of humor, looking on the bright side, being determined or strong, loving life, and enjoying little things. This is highly related to level of self-confidence. Religiousness and keeping busy are distant third and fourth. Some people mention emersion in nature as a way to put their troubles in perspective.

Spiritual development is one of the few goals that increase in importance with age. In my longitudinal study, for example, at the last data point in 1995 everyone was age 70 or older. Seventy-nine percent said that compared with when they were 50, their inner life was more important to them now. Spiritual development supports adaptation by fostering a perspective in which time becomes panoramic and space become infinite. In such a context, there is less to be anxious about.

Lars Tornstam (1994) developed the theory of gerotranscendence, which holds that as people age they gradually transcend the biological, psychological, and social bonds that cause us so much anxiety. In my longitudinal study, I found that compared with when they were 50, a large proportion of respondents said that they were less afraid of death now, felt a greater connection with the universe, and got more enjoyment from their inner life.

When we see elders just sitting, we are quick to assume that there is nothing going on, but we may be wrong. I had the following conversation with an 80-year-old woman:

"There are times when you seem to be in a far-off place in your mind," I said.

"Yes," she said.
"Is it a pleasant place," I asked.
"Oh my, yes," she said.
"Can you tell me what it is like," I asked.

She replied, "Words don't describe it. It's warm and cozy. Thoughts come and go, but are of no importance. I feel completely at peace."

No wonder she liked to have her contemplative time in the afternoons. We should be careful not to assume that everyone needs to be busy all the time. Contemplative time is important, too.

CHALLENGES TO COPING

Most elders live in a world in which continuity and spiritual development are robust resources for coping. However, two things can happen to make elders more vulnerable: disability and thinning of the social network. When this happens, continuity needs to be seen as evolutionary, not business as usual. With brittle continuity, elders try to maintain independence, often at the expense of social contact. Elders needing long-term care prefer to get it at home, but unless they have a very rich social network indeed, they may find themselves increasingly isolated.

Research shows that elders are constantly making new acquaintances and developing new friendships. But as people become home-bound this becomes much more difficult. Unless they are tied into a community with strong outreach, elders can find themselves in a situation where the only people they see are those who are paid to visit–often not a good situation.

Take the case of Mrs. E, who lived in a small city of 25,000 in the Midwestern U.S. At 65, she lived alone, but was very active in her community. She founded a singles group for middle-aged and older adults and was very active in state politics, often hosting visiting candidates and doing logistics for their events. She spent her time caring for her small home, flower arranging, and visiting with her many friends. She was also close to two older sisters who lived about an hour's drive away. Her life was full of activity, she found meaning in relationships, and also enjoyed her solitude.

At 75, Mrs. E had had a stroke, which left her balance impaired and required that she give up driving and use a three-wheeled walker to get around. Gradually she lost contact with many of her friends. They visited at first, but as the months went by they gradually stopped visiting.

Her sisters were also becoming more impaired and their visits became much less frequent, although they kept in touch by phone. Mrs. E required help with bathing, meal preparation, medication management, and housekeeping. She could no longer do flower arranging or decorating without assistance, and because getting out was so difficult, she became increasingly house-bound. Without the mental stimulation of being with others, Mrs. E became increasingly paranoid and became more and more fearful about new residents in the neighborhood and even the service providers who came to set up her medication trays or deliver meals. Her activities consisted of watching television, cooking an occasional meal, reading the newspaper, poring over catalogs, and talking with her sisters on the phone. She became increasingly isolated.

At 79, Mrs. E had another stroke, which was at least in part brought on by her inability to follow her medication regimen. She was worried about the expense of her medications and would save the medication instead of taking it. Her doctors did not expect her to survive this stroke, but she did. During her lengthy recovery, she lived in a nursing home near her daughter, who lived in an adjacent state. Gradually, she recovered her ability to speak and walk with a walker. Because she was in a rich social environment in the nursing home, she also recovered her excellent social skills and made many new friends. The art therapy staff person at the nursing home was very encouraging, and Mrs. E discovered an interest in watercolors. Some of her watercolors were featured in local exhibitions. The activities program at the nursing home offered her many opportunities to listen to musical performances, attend religious services, do her art, and keep up with current events—all things she had stopped doing when she was housebound.

Mrs. E and I had the following conversation about a year after her move to the nursing home.

"Do you miss [your former home and community]? I asked.
"Not really," she replied.
"Would you want to go back?"
"No."
"Why not," I asked.
"I like it here," she said.
"What's so special about here?"
"The people. I have lots of people to help me, I get to do a lot of things I enjoy, and I get to see [her daughter and son-in-law] more, and I can still talk to my sisters on the phone. I've made new friends. Art excites me."

At 80, Mrs. E seems much more contented with life than she did at 75. Her case illustrates how a supportive environment can help a person reconstitute continuity. Mrs. E's awakened interest in art is very much a new spiritual connection for her.

In working with elders, it is important to remember that most of them have two somewhat contradictory goals: remaining independent and maintaining their social network. Often, to maintain the social network means having to accept help both in getting out and in bringing people in. The need to be independent and self-reliant, which is so important to most people, can become a hindrance to good adaptation when disability occurs. Without help, everyday tasks of self-care become so energy- and time-intensive that they are all-consuming and leave little in the way of resources for elements that maintain quality of life. One way to work with this situation is to include social elements in care plans. Being in the flow of art or music is not an instrumental value, but it can nourish the soul. And both can have the advantage of not being dependent on verbal ability. Thus art and music are not just activities designed to keep people busy. They can also have spiritual and healing qualities.

Continuity theory can help us map the personal system of those we serve. By asking careful questions about what has been important to the person in the past, we can see how to help them see ways to realize their underlying values in the present. However, we cannot expect them to voluntarily turn their back on a life structure that has served them well in the past. That is why most people cannot see anything good about moving to an assisted living or nursing home setting. They need help in seeing continuity in their life before and after the move. Most fundamentally, continuity resides in the values that inform choice, not just in the specifics of everyday environments and activities.

CONCLUSION

I have painted an optimistic picture of aging and the human spirit based on my 35 years of research on adaptation to various aspects of aging. I have gained tremendous respect for the people I have studied, for their magnificent insights and capabilities. I also have great admiration for their capacity to prevail in the face of what sometimes seem insurmountable difficulties. My main points for you are that continuity of values, attitudes, lifestyles, and relationships as well as spiritual development in later adulthood provide most people with robust resources for coping with changing circumstances and also provide a sense of direction.

In order to be of help to elders, we can benefit from having a framework with which we can learn about their personal systems. Those who work with elders can use these perspectives to discover and support their clients' aspirations for the last stages of life.

Continuity and spiritual growth are robust resources that see most people through the aging process. But disability and the thinning of the social network can create a need to reconfigure the personal system. Many people need outreach services that accompany and support them as they modify their personal system to their new circumstances. Continuity and spiritual development are our friends in this process, too.

REFERENCES

Atchley, R. C. (1996) *The Journey*. A poem–copyright Atchley.

Atchley, R. C. (1999). *Continuity and adaptation in aging: Creating positive experiences.* Baltimore: John Hopkins University Press.

Atchley, R. C. (2000). Spirituality. In T.R. Cole et al. (Eds.), *Handbook of the humanities and aging* (2nd ed) (pp. 324-341). New York: Springer.

Atchley, R. C. (2003). Becoming a spiritual elder. In M.A. Kimble & S.H. McFadden (Eds.), *Aging, spirituality, and religion: A handbook* (Vol. 2) (pp. 33-46). Minneapolis: Fortress Press.

Atchley, R. C. (2004). *Serving from spirit.* www.servingfromspirit.com

Atchley, R. C. (2005). *The path of service in later adulthood.* Paper presented to the annual meeting of the American Society on Aging. Philadelphia, March 12.

Erikson, E. H., Erikson, J. M., & Kivnick, H. Q. (1986). *Vital involvement in old age.* New York: W. W. Norton.

Spiritual Eldering Institute (2004). *www.spiritualeldering.org*

Tornstam, L. (1994). Gerotranscendence: A theoretical and empirical exploration. In L. E. Thomas & S. A. Eisenhandler (Eds.), *Aging and the religious dimension* (pp. 203-229). New York: Auburn House.

The Spirituality of Compassion:
A Public Health Response to Ageing
and End-of-Life Care

Bruce Rumbold, MSc, PhD, BD (Hons), MA

SUMMARY. The recent revival of interest in spirituality in later life marks a significant step forward in the person-centred care of ageing people. The benefits will, however, be of limited value if we do not attend to the settings in which spirituality is to be lived. In contemporary society many aged people are located in environments unsympathetic to spiritual belief and practice. Health care settings focus on professionally-assessed physical needs and are dominated by concerns about the cost of services. The national social policies that direct health care services and less directly shape older people's place in contemporary society are strongly influenced by globalised neoliberal economic policies characterised by individualism, competition, and greed. For robust and viable spirituality to develop at the individual level we need compassionate social policies that support interdependence within communities and between nations. *[Article copies available for a fee from The Haworth Document Delivery Service: 1-800-HAWORTH. E-mail address: <docdelivery@ haworthpress.com> Website: <http://www.HaworthPress.com> © 2006 by The Haworth Press, Inc. All rights reserved.]*

Bruce Rumbold, MSc, PhD, BD (Hons), MA, is affiliated with the Palliative Care Unit, School of Public Health, La Trobe University, Melbourne, 3068, Australia.

[Haworth co-indexing entry note]: "The Spirituality of Compassion: A Public Health Response to Ageing and End-of-Life Care." Rumbold, Bruce. Co-published simultaneously in *Journal of Religion, Spirituality & Aging* (The Haworth Pastoral Press, an imprint of The Haworth Press, Inc.) Vol. 18, No. 2/3 , 2006, pp. 31-44; and: *Aging, Spirituality and Palliative Care* (ed: Elizabeth MacKinlay) The Haworth Pastoral Press, an imprint of The Haworth Press, Inc., 2006, pp. 31-44. Single or multiple copies of this article are available for a fee from The Haworth Document Delivery Service [1-800-HAWORTH, 9:00 a.m. - 5:00 p.m. (EST). E-mail address: docdelivery@haworthpress.com].

KEYWORDS. Ageing, compassion, globalization, public health, social policy, spirituality

Western societies have had less than fifty years' experience in living with a population profile that includes a large number of aged people. We've tried to deal with the situation using patterns that worked–after a fashion–with other social problems. We've focused on the changing bodies and minds of ageing people, seeing these as medical challenges to be overcome or contained. The gaze of health professionals has shaped social policy on ageing, and our responses have attended principally to clinical management problems and risk reduction concerns. It's not surprising that so far we've really only managed warehousing solutions for the 'problem' of the aged members of our population, storing them in institutions on the margins of our society.

In recent years, public health approaches have attempted to redress the negative perception of ageing that arises from this clinical management. New public health perspectives (Baum, 2004) emphasise constructive approaches to health, presenting it as more than the absence of disease and disability. Health is created in communities that appreciate the richness and diversity of human experience. A fundamental requirement for health is a healthy environment, for health is socially determined. And consequently public health strategies involve much more than the provision of 'health services': we need to develop healthy communities, healthy cities, and healthy societies.

A public health approach thus focuses on settings–personal, social, and physical environments–and the way these are shaped by social policy at the local and national levels to achieve healthy outcomes for populations. Health is seen as something too important to be left to health services, which are in practice largely illness services.

Public health strategies have the twin goals of preventing illness and creating health. If an illness or condition cannot be prevented, strategic interest turns to harm-minimisation. In either case, early intervention–addressing a situation before it becomes a pressing problem–is preferred. Because health is socially determined, both preventing illness and creating health involve changing settings or environments. Further, priority is given to strategies that are participatory–that work with, not on, communities–and sustainable, not indefinitely reliant on professional support, even if initially such support is required to facilitate change.

PUBLIC HEALTH AND SUCCESSFUL AGEING

The public health approach to aged care that moves beyond problem-based studies of ageing is only a recent phenomenon: for example, a health and well-being category of research appears for the first time in 1993 Australian directories (McCormack, 2000). Much of the focus of this work is upon harm-minimisation in the sense of finding ways of reducing the deleterious impacts of ageing–although some clinical gerontology programs appear to be interested in preventing ageing itself (Vincent, 2003). Social inclusion of ageing people is also a research priority (Tanner, 2001). In practice, however, successful ageing continues to be promoted as being able to keep doing the things that younger people do. Public health programs promoting successful ageing can thus paradoxically reinforce the stigma of ageism, and further marginalize those in the 'Fourth Age' who are for the most part highly vulnerable (Baltes & Smith, 2003). As we shall see later in this discussion, the messages of successful ageing are continually undercut by contrary messages from social and economic policy.

For ageing to escape being solely a health management problem we need still broader views of health that can incorporate being as well as doing, dying as well as living. And here is the nub of the problem. The disciplines of public health and gerontology share a reluctance to face death. For both, avoiding death is the primary motivation for adopting healthy behaviours. In this respect the new public health is very much like the older versions that promoted clinical medicine. But such avoidance of death is neither necessary nor beneficial, and taking account of spirituality may be a way forward.

SPIRITUALITY RETURNS TO HEALTH DISCOURSE

Spirituality, a major theme in traditional understandings of health, has re-appeared in recent discourse as health disciplines venture to consider possibilities in the face of death or permanent disability. Admittedly, spirituality is frequently invoked as a stop-gap solution when chronic illness and degenerative illness have become intractable from a medical perspective. Not surprisingly, in modern times palliative care was the first discipline to give formal acknowledgement to spirituality as a resource in caring for dying people. Palliative care attracted the support and interest it did because it revived the concept of a good death for deaths that were 'out of time,' deaths from cancer of people who had failed to attain old age.

Only recently has a palliative approach begun to consider the question of a good death in old age, usually by invoking ideas of completing a spiritual journey. Spirituality allows people to cope with the diminishment and dependence of old age and make a good end to their lives (MacKinlay, 2001). Even so, most of these discussions of spirituality limit themselves to the spiritual experience and needs of aged individuals. The argument in this paper is that, in addition to this individual focus, sometimes even instead of it, attention needs to be paid to the spirituality of the settings in which these older people are located. Many of these settings resist attending to spirituality at all, and some of those that are interested in spirituality espouse approaches that may not meet the needs of ageing people.

To explore these ideas further I will turn to a schematic social history of old age, which will indicate that today's narratives about ageing are not the only options offered by our culture. I'll present this in terms of the major forms of social organization that have characterized Western society to this point (Walter, 1994), which can be labelled Traditional, Modern and Contemporary. The first two terms are generally accepted, while the third continues to be debated. Contemporary social organization has been identified variously as late modernity, high modernity, reflexive modernity, neo-modernity, and post-modernity. What seems clear is that we are moving beyond modern forms, and that what we are to become has not yet been revealed. We live at present in a society that displays both traditional and modern characteristics, but is distinctive in the way it draws upon and blends these influences.

Each form of social organization offers its own understanding of human identity and human community. Thus ageing, and spirituality, are viewed differently in each era. The key characteristics of these frameworks are in Table 1.

Many contemporary ideas about ageing and spirituality, containing statements about the dignity and wisdom of age, sound as if they have been drawn from traditional religious society; but these are in reality fragments of what they once were. Themes that were shared social beliefs of the past, reflected in social practices, have been reduced to ideas that may be held by some individuals. While traditional values concerning ageing have a lingering resonance in our society, they contribute more to social rhetoric than social policy.

Far more influential in shaping the social experience of ageing people are the shifts in social identity that have overtaken all who live in

TABLE 1

Form of social organization	TRADITIONAL	MODERN	CONTEMPORARY
Technology	Pre-industrial	Industrial	Globalised communication networks
Central authority	Religion	Science	Self
Social structures	Hierarchical: based on custom & inheritance	Knowledge-based	Blending traditional and modern forms: continually negotiated
Health	Subordinate to salvation	Absence of disease	Expressing the whole person
Spirituality	Led by religious specialists	Private concern of religious individuals	Focuses on the human spirit: complex relationship with religion
Identity	Through community: the people to whom you belong	Through production: the work that you do	Through the body: how you present yourself
Elderly people	A minority: care depends on the benevolence of others	Increasing in number: care provided through government welfare programs	Significant proportion of population: care is each individual's responsibility
Good death	Religiously determined	Private	Self-determined

contemporary late modern societies. For young adults, whose identities have been formed in the midst of the transition from modern to late modern organization, the effects may be minimal. But for elderly people, whose identities were formed in the modern era, the shifts can be confusing and disabling. Having been raised to think of themselves as producers contributing through their labour to the common good, they are now invited to understand themselves as consumers. Having lived their adult lives as citizens expecting to receive retirement benefits in due recognition of their contribution to society, they find themselves purchasers of services they had expected to receive by right, as pensions give way to superannuation and what were previously entitlements become their personal responsibility (Wilson, 2002). Even the idea of a natural decline as age increases–the life cycle model–has been replaced by a life span idea in which they are expected to demonstrate 'successful ageing' for as long as possible.

In apparent contradiction to these messages, aged people may find themselves the object of alarmism and scape-goating from politicians who wish to further ideological goals of reducing government expenditure on welfare. They will become used to being portrayed as an actual or potential burden and consequently a threat to the financial security of their children and grandchildren. They may find their anticipated rights and activities curtailed for the sake of equity (Phillipson, 1998). Old age is increasingly 'reconstructed as a phase in life negotiated by the individual, rather than an experience controlled by and developed through mass institutions such as the welfare state' (Phillipson, 2003, Para 2.4).

SPIRITUALITY AND AGEING

Can spirituality be a resource that supports aged people in such sustained attacks upon their expectations and self-understanding? For some no doubt it will be, allowing them to resist the ambivalent cultural messages surrounding them and to continue finding meaning and purpose in their lives. For others, this ambivalence will undermine the spirituality that has nurtured them in the past, or that spirituality will falter because today's communities no longer support their particular forms of belief and practice.

As already noted above, spirituality too has changed. Framed in modern times as an individual's choice of particular religious practices, spirituality takes on a different shape in contemporary society. It attends less to ideas about God as a spiritual being who calls out a response in us, God's creatures, than it does to the mystery of the human spirit. Thus today to assert my spirituality may not be to name my allegiance to a religious position so much as to claim my unique individual identity. My spirituality is my achievement and uniquely defines who I am. In the name of spirituality I celebrate my distinctiveness and resist the attempts of others to prescribe my beliefs about myself. The content will be more about who I am than about who God–or any higher power– might be. And because this social understanding of spirituality shapes the understanding of many in the contemporary church, religious practice may not provide the spiritual support many older people had hoped for. Needing spiritual support that focuses on right practice and right belief–the traditional and modern emphases–they may find themselves invited to construct a spirituality that is the right fit for them, or to embrace experiential approaches that are unfamiliar to them. Some may welcome these approaches, but others may find them wanting.

Spirituality is not, however, solely an attribute or possession of an individual so much as it describes the set of relationships that connect that individual to self, the social world, and the environment. While the details of these relationships are unique to each individual, the pattern they assume is not. Lartey (1997, p. 113) suggests, for example, that spirituality involves relationships:

- With places and things (spatial)
- With self (intra-personal)
- With others (inter-personal)
- Among people (corporate)
- With transcendence

Spirituality is that which gives coherence to this web or system of connections that link people into life. Spirituality may be represented, and accessed, through objects, places, rituals, reflection, relationships, beliefs–but it is not limited to any of these. Maintaining and nurturing spirituality will involve paying attention to the full range of connections, not just those that fall into the category of 'beliefs' or inner work (Rumbold, 2002). And because those connections link us with aspects of a changing world, our spirituality continues to be influenced by the spirituality–the connections and implicit values–of our setting. Conceptualising spirituality in this way can help in understanding both the problems people face in maintaining spiritual practice in aversive environments, and ways in which attention to settings might sustain and nurture spiritual practice.

SPIRITUALITY AND SETTINGS

In modern and late modern times spirituality is generally attributed to individuals. But my argument here is that spirituality is strongly linked with individuals' responses to the setting in which they find themselves, not just with an inner life that might be maintained because or in spite of the setting. A particular setting assumes and reinforces a set of values, evoking certain spiritualities and challenging others (Pembroke, 2004). Thus spirituality intersects with social policy.

The connection between spirituality and settings can be linked with the concept of the 'hidden curriculum,' illustrated for example by Westerhoff's (1976) discussion of the schooling-instruction paradigm of learning. Schools in the era in which he was writing–and even more so today–were required to instruct students on equal opportunity. Such formal instruction was made available in the classrooms, but the informal learning was very different. As he pointed out in observing one school, while female teachers went into both boys' and girls' rooms, male teachers only went into boys' rooms; girls and boys were encouraged to play very different sorts of games; teachers corrected or punished boys and girls in very different ways; there were no male kindergarten teachers and no female administrators; photographs in the classrooms reinforced these role divisions. How effective, he asked, could a training course expect to be in the face of contradictory learning from this hidden curriculum?

While there may have been some movement in the schooling-instruction paradigm in recent decades, our health systems still frequently place themselves in *loco parentis* to infantilised elders. Kitwood's description (1997, p. 46-7) of what he called the malignant social psychology of dementia care institutions is a graphic example of this. He asserted that many such institutions were characterised by:

> Treachery, Infantilisation, Labelling, Outpacing, Banishment, Ignoring, Withholding, Disruption, Disempowerment, Intimidation, Stigmatisation, Invalidation, Objectification, Imposition, Accusation, Mockery, Disparagement. (Kitwood, 1997, pp. 46-7)

The effect, he claimed–and was able to demonstrate–is that a dementing person removed from such a setting is capable of re-menting. The spirituality of the setting dominates that of the individuals within it, limiting their already-reduced social roles and diffusing further their fragile sense of self.

Independent living in the community is prized until health problems emerge, at which point the system steps in and may take over your life. The risks you were able to take in living independently are unacceptable in a system that sees itself responsible for your welfare at all times and liable for any accident that might befall you. The alternative to independence is, apparently, complete dependence. There are, encouragingly, some signs that this issue is being addressed through concepts like 'the dignity of risk' (Nay, 2002). Nay concludes that 'overzealous risk management may protect a physical body from bruising but it may also damage irreparably the already vulnerable human soul' (2002, p. 33). But the ageism and risk management that characterize the health system are reasons why many elderly people avoid seeking assistance in the first place (Minichiello et al., 2000). Frequently an inability to be self-reliant leads to reduced self-esteem and loss of purpose in life, largely because of the way services are provided. In contrast, Secker et al. (2003) show that it is possible to combine high levels of (physical) dependence with high levels of experienced independence if aged people are involved in planning care in ways that maintain self-determination and preserve a sense of continuity in life.

Many of the problems outlined above stem from welfare approaches to aged care. It is assumed that aged people will become an increasing burden upon the state both through expanding health care costs and the need for the state to supply supported residential care. While this assumption holds for only a limited number of aged people, the institutionalisation of some colours social attitudes to the many.

THE IMPACT OF GLOBALISATION

Globalisation opposes these welfare approaches and has accelerated the late modern changes to social identity outlined above. Globalisation denotes a new integration of social, economic and political systems, made possible by new means of transport and communication, but this is an interdependence driven by capital. The logic of globalisation is that capital is accountable primarily to shareholders, and only in partial ways to the nation-states that are responsible for the health and welfare of their citizens (Wilson, 2002). The growing influence of global capital, exercised both through the markets and agencies such as the World Bank and the International Monetary Fund, reduces the role of the state to that of funding and promoting market solutions and placing greater responsibility upon individuals for their own welfare (Estes & Phillipson, 2002).

Globalisation offers the possibility of constructive reform of the welfare systems that can construct unhealthy dependence, but as globalisation operates today it provides options only for those with wealth. Further, that wealth is developed and maintained at the expense of the poorest (Rapley, 2004). Longevity is itself an indicator of global inequality, for it is the product of societies that monopolise the world's resources: that is, it's a phenomenon for the 15% of the world population that isn't part of a minority ethnic or socio-economic group and lives in North America, Europe, Australasia, or Japan. In general, globalisation as an economic ideology compromises health, particularly in developing nations. As Awafeso notes:

> Poor nation-states, and poor communities within rich nation-states—
> who are already at risk locally from inadequate water, poor sani-

tation, and inadequate food–are faced with a "double burden" of adverse environmental and health conditions as multinational industries relocate to such societies. (2002, p. 137)

Shareholder risk of reduced profits is thereby minimized, but in effect this risk is exported to heighten the health risks of poor nation-states and of those who lose employment in the more affluent society from which the industry departs. Our anxieties about our own ageing help to drive this cycle, for superannuation investment funds are major players in the market. The search for profits large enough to fund our many retirement years reduces life expectancy elsewhere. The market is characterized by competition, anxiety, self-interest, and greed.

PROMOTING INTERDEPENDENCE

If globalization is inimical to health, are there alternatives? The short answer is yes. While economic development is a desirable goal, particularly for poor countries, the pursuit of economic development does not have to mean the neglect of all priorities other than materialist ones. As Michael Edwards puts it:

Inequalities result from political decisions about the distribution of gains from economic activity. What is allocated to private consumption, public spending and social responsibilities is never fixed, and it is democracy's job–not the role of markets–to determine our collective goals and common interests. (Edwards, 2001, p. 385)

Edwards argues that capital must be humanized, which, among other things, will involve a return to an acknowledged interdependence that goes beyond mere economics, or at least starts to place monetary value on things that matter. Senator Robert Kennedy once famously remarked that the GNP (Gross National Product) measures everything except that which makes life worthwhile. Edwards points out that there 'can't be much sense in a system that . . . counts weapons production on a par with investment in schools, treats child care as valueless, and discounts the cost of pollution' (2001, p. 393). Valuing interdependence is, however, resisted by neoliberal economic ideology because, Twine (1994) asserts, doing so 'would present us with moral obligations to compensate those who bear the costs of our progress' (1994, p. 29).

Nevertheless, addressing inequality makes good sense even at a materialist level. As Eckersley (2002) points out, the evidence is that life expectancy rises with per capita income at lower income levels, but among rich nations is only weakly related to average income, and may even begin to decline as the growing social inequality associated with affluence precipitates poorer health outcomes. Research suggests that increasing equality in affluent nations like Australia would do more for population health than increasing the average income.

THE SPIRITUALITY OF COMPASSION

Promoting interdependence requires us to listen to older people's perceptions and experiences and to challenge the dominance of policies dictated by particular market ideologies. This in turn requires social structures that recognize these tasks as twin aspects of the same ethical imperative. Recognising the rights of marginalized groups to be heard and resisting the forces that marginalize and silence them will come about if compassion is an ethical imperative in developing social policy (Kellehear, 2005).

Compassion is a core value of interdependence. A number of recent theories of care have been built around the concept of love, but the problem with this is that multiple meanings render the term capable of being individualised, sentimentalised, or abused. Compassion aligns itself with *agape* from amongst these multiple meanings of love. It is universal and inclusive, a core concept for a range of religious traditions and spiritual practices. It links empathy, understanding and justice, promoting inter-dependence.

> To train in compassion is to know that all beings are the same and suffer in similar ways, to honour all those that suffer, and to know that you are neither separate from nor superior to anyone. (Soygal Rinpoche, 1992)

As spiritual care invites us to build mutual human relationships and create receptive spaces, rather than to make assessments and deliver interventions, our fundamental task becomes that of creating compassionate settings. This involves us in revisioning care. Liz Lloyd reminds us that care is a central concern for all human beings, which includes the need not only *for* care but *to* care (Lloyd, 2004, p. 247). Our social understandings of care can no longer afford to be shaped by clinical practice that presents care as a paid activity dominated by risk management procedures. And to re-evaluate risk management approaches we need to change our understanding of risk. This necessitates moving from 'capital' as a measure of worth to 'social capital.' Social capital approaches value cooperation for mutual benefit, community participation and support, trust and respect, and the interaction of communities, including those communities that have been marginalised under the reign of capital alone (Fine, 2001). Social capital values that which makes life worthwhile in a way that capital alone has notoriously failed to do.

Investing in social transformation will require significant shifts in all modern institutions, including churches. Judging from the way in which church financial resources are increasingly tied up in maintaining and staffing worship facilities, churches may need to choose between conserving these structures and creating new communities. It would be a major step for churches to support social capital development by selling up worship facilities, but the social evidence is that worship facilities have failed to transform society, while new approaches to community might.

A social capital approach also requires us to manage globalisation rather than have it manage us. This has implications, for example, for all of us who invest, as we are obliged to, in superannuation funds. An imperative for fund choice needs to be ethical investment. Otherwise our anxieties about ageing will continue to drive the competition that maximizes profits and sabotages the possibilities of others. In turn this requires us to find our life other than in possessions. We need to acknowledge interdependence, to practise relinquishment of some of our financial expectations, in pursuit of a vision for a world in which health, justice and constructive longevity are accessible to all. Only then will we be able to articulate the nature of social justice and rights for those who depend on others for support and care. At present these concepts are inextricably linked with independence and autonomy, and those who in later life become physically dependent must "depend also upon the moral orientation of others for their well-being" (Lloyd, 2004, p. 236).

CONCLUSION

To attend to each individual's spirituality, particularly in health care and aged care settings, is admirable. But this approach will be ineffectual or even counter-productive if it is not matched by attention to the way social settings nurture, or more frequently fail to nurture, the spirituality of those who participate in them. It has been argued here that contemporary social policy in significant respects opposes spiritual values and thereby undermines spiritual growth. Further development in the spiritual care of individuals can only continue through wide-ranging changes in social values. We need in particular to recognise that care–giving and receiving–is at the centre of human experience, and that compassion is an ethical imperative for human societies. This ethical stance invites us to reframe globalisation in terms of social capital, and social policy in terms of interdependence.

REFERENCES

Awafeso, N. (2002). Letter to the editor: Globalisation and health. *NSW Public Health Bulletin 13, 6*, 137-8.

Baltes, P., & Smith, J. (2003). New frontiers in the future of aging: From successful aging of the young/old to the dilemmas of the fourth age. *Gerontology 49, 2*, 123-135.

Baum, F. (2004). *The new public health: An Australian perspective.* Melbourne: Oxford University Press.

Eckersley, R. (2002). Health, well-being, and progress. *NSW Public Health Bulletin 13, 6*, 128-130.

Edwards, M. (2001). Humanising global capitalism: Which way forward? In A. Giddens (Ed.), *The global third way debate,* 384-393. Cambridge: Polity Press.

Estes, C., & Phillipson, C. (2002). The globalization of capital, the welfare state, and old age policy. *International Journal of Health Services 32, 2*, 279-297.

Fine, B. (2001). *Social capital versus social theory.* London: Routledge.

Kellehear, A. (2005). *Compassionate cities: Public health and end-of-life care.* London: Routledge.

Kitwood, T. (1997). *Dementia reconsidered: The person comes first.* Buckingham: Open University Press.

Lartey, E. (1997). *In living colour: An intercultural approach to pastoral care and counselling.* London: Cassell.

Lloyd, L. (2004). Mortality and morality: Ageing and the ethics of care. *Ageing and Society 24*, 235-256.

McCormack, J. (2000). Looking back and moving forward? Ageing in Australia 2000. *Ageing and Society 20*, 623-631.

MacKinlay, E. (2001). *The spiritual dimension of ageing.* London: Jessica Kingsley.

Minichiello, V., Browne, J., & Kendig, H. (2000). Perceptions and consequences of ageism: The views of older people. *Ageing and Society 20*, 253-278.

Nay, R. (2002). The dignity of risk. *Australian Nursing Journal 9, 9*, 33.

Pembroke, N. (2004). *Working relationships: Spirituality in human service and organizational life.* London: Jessica Kingsley.

Phillipson, C. (1998). *Reconstructing old age: New agendas in social theory and practice.* London: Sage.

Phillipson, C. (2003). Globalisation and the future of ageing: Developing a critical gerontology. *Sociological Research Online 8*, 4. *http://www.socresoline.org.uk/8/4/phillipson.
   html*

Rapley, J. (2004). *Globalization and inequality: Neoliberalism's downward spiral.* Boulder: Lynne Rienner Publishers.

Rinpoche, S. (1992). *The Tibetan book of living and dying.* San Francisco: Harper San
   Francisco.

Rumbold. B. (Ed.) (2002). *Spirituality and palliative care: Social and pastoral perspectives.* Melbourne: Oxford University Press.

Secker, J., Hill, R., Villeneau, L., & Parkman, S. (2003). Promoting independence: But
   promoting what and how? *Ageing and Society 23*, 375-391.

Tanner, D. (2001). Sustaining the self in later life: Supporting older people in community. *Ageing & Society 21*, 255-278.

Twine, F. (1994). *Citizenship and social rights: The interdependence of self and society.*
   Thousand Oaks: Sage.

Vincent, J. (2003). What is at stake in the "War on anti ageing medicine"? *Ageing and
   Society 23*, 675-684.

Walter, T. (1994). *The revival of death.* London: Routledge.

Westerhoff, J. (1976). *Will our children have faith?* Melbourne: Dove Communications.

Wilson, G. (2002). Globalisation and older people: Effects of markets and migration.
   Ageing and Society 22, 647-663.

Disembodied Souls or Soul-Less Bodies: Spirituality as Fragmentation

Rosalie Hudson, RN, MTh, PhD

SUMMARY. 'Soul' and 'body' are two linguistic expressions of one and the same reality, the human being. In pastoral care, aged care, and palliative care the stated aim is always to care for the whole person. An increasing focus on 'spirituality' has also led to objectifying and measuring what is ultimately beyond calculation. To care for each person as an 'ensouled body' and 'embodied soul' is to acknowledge we are in the service of one another. In entering one another's stories, words like impose, define, and manage are replaced by trust, love, and faithfulness. Measurable outcomes are then replaced by risk, ambiguity, and mystery: the heart and soul and body of human care. *[Article copies available for a fee from The Haworth Document Delivery Service: 1-800-HAWORTH. E-mail address: <docdelivery@haworthpress.com> Website: <http://www.HaworthPress.com> © 2006 by The Haworth Press, Inc. All rights reserved.]*

KEYWORDS. Spirituality, palliative care, aged care, pastoral care, embodied soul, ensouled body, love, faithfulness

Rosalie Hudson, RN, MTh, PhD, is Associate Professor (Honorary Principal Fellow), School of Nursing, University of Melbourne, Aged Care/Palliative Care Consultant, PO Box 585, Northcote 3070, Victoria, Australia (E-mail: rhudson@websurf.net.au).

[Haworth co-indexing entry note]: "Disembodied Souls or Soul-Less Bodies: Spirituality as Fragmentation." Hudson, Rosalie. Co-published simultaneously in *Journal of Religion, Spirituality & Aging* (The Haworth Pastoral Press, an imprint of The Haworth Press, Inc.) Vol. 18, No. 2/3 , 2006, pp. 45-57; and: *Aging, Spirituality and Palliative Care* (ed: Elizabeth MacKinlay) The Haworth Pastoral Press, an imprint of The Haworth Press, Inc., 2006, pp. 45-57. Single or multiple copies of this article are available for a fee from The Haworth Document Delivery Service [1-800-HAWORTH, 9:00 a.m. - 5:00 p.m. (EST). E-mail address: docdelivery@haworthpress.com].

Available online at http://www.haworthpress.com/web/JRSA
© 2006 by The Haworth Press, Inc. All rights reserved.
doi:10.1300/J078v18n02_04

INTRODUCTION

Three examples set the scene for exploring the theme 'disembodied souls or soul-less bodies: spirituality as fragmentation.' First, in a discussion with a group of postgraduate palliative care nurses from a variety of practice settings, only three could state with confidence that they and their team integrated spirituality into their holistic care of patients and families. For some in the group, spiritual care was declared to be irrelevant to their practice; for others it was considered a purely private matter. For those who took the view that these matters were private, it followed that any disclosure from patient to nurse that sounded remotely 'spiritual' should remain confidential and, accordingly, should not be documented. It is ironic that the same nurses have no qualms at all about inquiring into their patients' intimate sexual history, or recording in detail their patients' bowel excretions, or carefully documenting their patients' highly individual and personal responses to pain. While all of the students agreed that palliative care is holistic care, it was evident that spiritual care was neither well understood nor widely practiced. Spirituality was generally regarded as being remote from bodily needs. A more integrated view of spirituality would acknowledge the inherent overlap of spiritual and physical, precisely when dealing with such matters as sex, bowels, and pain.

The second example comes from the United Kingdom, where a recent study in residential aged care homes found a much broader understanding of spirituality. When asked to rank various activities according to the criteria for spiritual care, respondents included the following: taking a resident on a trip to the countryside, enabling a resident to watch a particular TV program, and accompanying a resident on a walk in the garden. Also high on the list was comforting a resident who was worried about her incontinence. Staff clearly saw that addressing spiritual issues, however interpreted, was clearly their responsibility (Orchard & Clark, 2001). This study shows an integrated approach to care that acknowledges the spiritual/physical overlap.

The third example shows the imprecise nature of spirituality and the difficulty in locating its context. The story is told of a student nurse who asked her supervisor where she could 'find something on spirituality.' The supervisor responded impatiently, 'Look it up in the nurses' dictionary! You'll find it somewhere between sexuality and swallowing!'

Where does spirituality fit in holistic care? How is spiritual care distinguished from emotional, psychological and social care? Where does religion fit into this framework? Have we so broadened the concept of spirituality in our endeavour to divorce it from religion that we're left with nothing other than existential questions to be addressed by any humanist? What is being lost when we throw the religious baby out with the spiritual bathwater? Here, the words 'religion' and 'religious' are used to signify the Christian religion, not to deliberately ignore the many other religions in our pluralistic society, but to place the body/ soul subject matter within a Judeo-Christian biblical understanding.

In this paper, three major questions are raised, which will invariably overlap throughout the discussion. First, has the new spirituality pushed religion to the margins? Second, has 'spirit' language been overtaken by 'systemspeak,' and third, what happens to our humanity when we separate soul from body?

Soul and Body

'Soul' and 'body' are two linguistic expressions of one and the same reality, the human being. Computerized tomography reveals in precise detail more and more about the body but it cannot map, scan, locate, describe, or explain the soul. Any attempt to label or categorise the indefinable 'soul' apart from 'body' is fraught with profound difficulties, as Cobb indicates:

> We can say that the body is life, that which is alive, and that the soul is what enlivens or animates. Yet both are so profoundly interrelated that every attempt to objectify either of them without the other in the end leads to absurdity. (Cobb, 2001, p. 70)

Soul is not a self-contained entity. Here, we struggle against the Cartesian legacy that separated the mind from the body and science from theology. Descartes (1586-1650) gave the human body a mechanical description but he did not completely ignore the soul (after all, he attended Mass every Sunday and his first name was Emanual!), but the only way he could incorporate the soul was to regard it as an anatomical structure, locating it in the pineal gland of the brain (Stumpf, 1994, p. 249). For Descartes, we are human beings because our rational capacity makes us so. 'I think, therefore I am.' Damasio reverses Descartes' ordering when he states 'We are, and then we think' (Damasio, 1994, p. 248).

In this discussion, Descartes' dictum is given a further twist, based on the premise that we are human beings, not in isolation, but in relationship with each other: 'We are in community, therefore we *are*' (Hudson, 2004). As well as being philosophically locked into the Enlightenment legacy that separates soul from body, we remain in a Platonic prison when we regard the human being as *composed* of *a* soul and *a* body (Tarazi, 1999, p. 76). For Plato the soul was 'divine' and thus immortal, while the body was merely the external casing bound for corruption. If we turn from Plato and Descartes to the Judeo-Christian scriptures we find immortality belongs to God alone (1 Tim 6: 16) and our hope for eternal life lies not in the immortality of our souls as separate entities but in the resurrection of our *bodies, who we are as persons*, a point to be taken up later in the discussion.

To further illustrate the unity of body and soul let us consider the expressions 'there is not a soul in sight' or 'what is the body count?' These are not disembodied souls or soul-less bodies we're referring to; in both cases we mean human beings. Whether we use the word 'soul' or 'spirit' the Scriptures make it clear that we do not *have* a soul or spirit; rather, spirit is breathed into us at creation (Tarazi, 1999, p. 76). God breathes into the clay and man becomes a living soul. This is quite clearly not a body-less soul, as Anderson points out:

> The human spirit does not merely reside in the body as in a container, but becomes the life of the body. . . . The soul is not an indestructible core of our being, which somehow survives our physical death. Both body and soul are who we are as mortal beings. . . . (Anderson, 2003, p. 169)

For St. Paul, soul and body are not synonyms for spiritual and unspiritual: the soul being the pure unsullied part of humanity while the body is the weak, sinful 'flesh.' Rather, 'spirit' and 'body' signify a sharing in the life God has given us; that life is quite clearly our *bodily, spirit-filled* life. For Karl Barth, the language that best describes our distinctive character as human beings is 'embodied souls' and 'besouled bodies' (Barth, 1960, pp. 350-352). The language of 'embodied soul' is also making an appearance in the nursing literature (Picard, 1997), in an attempt to recognise the fracturing of the human person that results from a false bifurcation of body and soul.

To reduce the spirit to a mere component part is to turn it into a problem waiting to happen. For example, the website for Palliative Care Australia refers to 'spiritual problems that are present with a terminal illness' (Palliative Care Australia). While the intent is to remind the reader that palliative care is holistic, the reference can be construed as artificially isolating the spirit, turning it into a problem. To spot a problem is (especially for nurses) to try to solve it. So, the logical consequence is to adopt the language of diagnosis, flow-charts, processes, pathways, goals, measurements, and outcomes, using engineering terms such as tools and instruments and other 'technospeak' for the profound mystery that is the human person.

While I plead guilty to developing a spiritual assessment form with the aim of trying to capture the elusive concept of spirituality in aged care, I also take seriously Walter's rebuke: 'The great spiritual teachers of the world would surely turn in their graves to hear spirituality turned into a discourse of clients, needs, goals, interventions, care plans, and outcomes!'(Walter, 1997). The problem with assessment forms is that they are so often put in the hands of staff that lack the necessary sensitivity, maturity, experience, and professionalism to use them wisely; they are also treated as a prompt sheet for interrogation rather than the basis for ongoing discussion. Spirituality emerges through a relationship of trust and respect, with an intimate connection to each person's life story. Disclosure may therefore consist of fragments over time, rather than a cohesive uninterrupted narrative. Spirituality is not a diagnostic category based on facts to be processed; spirituality involves the story of the person's life, which may, of course, never be fully told (Cobb & Robshaw, 1998, pp. 108-110).

Is there another way to reach the human person in his or her body/ spirit unity than to quickly grab a digging tool, or to search for the perfect instrument that will provide an inviolable measurement that will comply with the inescapable auditing requirements that will qualify us for the highest funding, that will help us to provide the spiritual care, that will further justify our systems in our well-meaning attempt to provide holistic care? This is not to suggest we do away with all spiritual assessment in whatever form (or forms). Rather, we should ask ourselves what is the best way to discover the essence of each particular person in our care, and to find a way of documenting the continuity of that unique life narrative. If we see the soul or spirit as a separate entity, particularly as the most private of all a person's 'private parts,' we will not be characters in the final chapter of that person's life story; we will merely be custodial caretakers of a physical body. If we enter the stories of those entrusted to our care we will see spirituality in its bodily reality, the 'real stuff' of ageing, death, and dying.

RELIGION PUSHED TO THE MARGINS

In pastoral care, aged care and palliative care the stated aim is always to care for the whole person. One of the hallmarks of palliative care is the interdisciplinary team and one of the great strengths of this teamwork lies in the sharing of responsibilities. However, not all team members have the expertise to offer symptom management for physical problems such as pain or vomiting; a volunteer, for example, would be expected to refer to the team member with the relevant professional expertise. Spiritual care, however, is becoming the province of the whole team. Whereas the first hospice declared in its *Aims and Basis:* 'St. Christopher's Hospice is based on the full Christian faith in God, through Christ' (Cobb & Robshaw, 1998, p. 170), today, 'palliative care's ambivalence about religion is reflected in the changing personnel involved in spiritual care' (Rumbold, 2002, p. 6).

Contemporary writers in this area, such as Cobb and Rumbold, are helping us to question what is happening here, particularly as we care for people approaching death.

> Not everything that takes place under the banner of palliative care needs to be carried out by professionals, but it seems reasonable to consider that the spiritual dimension of humanity is a sufficient weighty matter in the face of death to require considerable care and the utmost caution. (Cobb, 2001, p. 130)

In the aged care context the luxury of the multidisciplinary team is not formally evident (Hudson & Richmond, 2000, pp. 8-9), so there is even more likelihood that spiritual matters will be overlooked. Furthermore, the secular nature of contemporary society promotes a generic, 'religiously neutral' approach to spirituality that permeates the management structures of many residential aged care services (Hudson, 2003). This leaves residents without access to specific religious rituals and practices. However, the new guidelines for a palliative approach in residential aged care indicate a fresh pathway to best practice in spiritual care, including an increased emphasis on employing qualified, experienced chaplains (Commonwealth of Australia, 2004, p. 133). This does not necessarily mean all spiritual care is left to the chaplain. 'While chaplains have a unique role, spiritual care is enacted by all who care, through touch, gesture, even hesitant and clumsy words which convey the healing gift of one person's presence to another' (Hudson & Richmond, 2000, p. 138). It does mean that in any care context, health professionals should be able to discern when the patient has particular and specific religious needs to be addressed within the more generally defined spiritual framework.

'DUMBING DOWN' AND 'SYSTEMSPEAK'

In whatever context we are familiar with–aged care, palliative care, and pastoral care–we are confronted with a changing emphasis on spirituality, which I am suggesting is, in most cases, now so broad that it lacks any specificity at all. With so much emphasis on the spirit we may well wonder where the body went, particularly when the spirit is confined to an untouchable, ethereal realm. In a chapter called 'Dumbing down the spirit,' Pattison refers to 'floating spiritualities' which he describes as 'metaphysical marshmallow that is non-specific, unlocated, thin, uncritical, dull, and un-nutritious. Pastoral care which transmutes into generic spiritual care may become a case of the bland leading the bland' (Pattison, 2001, p. 34). In our attempt to embrace spirituality in its broadest connotations we may miss the precise focus that is needed. In our attempt to include spirituality in our plans of care we are in danger of adopting unhelpful bureaucratic language.

In the rapidly emerging spirituality literature (Baldacchino & Draper, 2001), sadly much of the language is 'systemspeak,' full of 'spiritual coping strategies' and 'spiritual orientation inventories,' not to mention double blind randomised control trials for measuring the effectiveness of prayer, and Likert scales for calculating belief. The new religionless spirituality has, in effect, become another 'religion,' reviving the ancient heresy of Gnosticism. [Although Gnosticism takes many forms, in this context it is used to refer to the first century 'special knowledge' by which a person's spiritual redemption protected them from all things related to the body or the 'material' world. Associated with this teaching was the belief that Jesus Christ was not truly human, but belonged only to the 'spiritual' world (Cross, 1997, p. 684).]

Unfortunately, when the separation of spirit from body is taken as dogma, it leads to the desire for control: objectifying, defining, intervening, categorizing, and measuring what is ultimately the mystery of human longing. Once we've diagnosed spiritual ills, then of course we have to prescribe a remedy, incorporating more 'system' language. But, as MacKinlay reminds us, there is no 'quick fix'; spiritual strategies are not 'pills that can be taken to cure a condition . . . but rather looking at issues that lie at the heart of what it is to be human' (MacKinlay, 2004, p. 75). Two examples serve as illustrations of this human care.

SPIRITUAL CARE IS HUMAN CARE

In her book of great wisdom and practical application, Shamy, a New Zealand Methodist minister, describes her first visit as pastoral carer to a day centre for people with dementia:

> The staff person introduced me to a room of silent men and women, totally lost within themselves. There was absolutely no response until I asked to be introduced personally to each person. I was taken to a seemingly lost and unaware old lady. 'Eileen, this is Ethel.' And quite spontaneously I exclaimed, 'Oh, Ethel. Ethel is the name of my mother-in-law.' What a transformation. Suddenly Ethel was sitting up straight, eyes bright and with a smile that I am sure started in her toes, for I saw it encompass her whole body until it reached her face and she stretched out her arms to embrace me, saying, 'Oh, my dear, we're related! We're related!' Then, with her eyes she gathered everyone in that room into our meeting, calling to them, 'We're related. We're related.' We were away–'related.' Related in our common humanity, related in our singing and our talking–all together–and, wonder, of wonders, in our dancing! (Shamy, 2003, p. 130)

Ethel, classified (for funding purposes no doubt) as cognitively impaired, shows remarkable insight by her spirited physical reaction. Eileen's response equally shows no fragmentation; body and spirit are one. As frequently happens, the patient becomes our teacher; or, as Goldsworthy's ministry with the frail elderly shows, many of those being ministered to are 'icons of grace' (Goldsworthy, 2003).

In his autobiography, Cochrane (of the Cochrane Collaboration on evidence based care) tells of his experience as medical officer in a German prisoner of war camp for Russians. The Germans had delivered a young Soviet prisoner to Cochrane's ward late at night.

> The ward was full, so I put him in my room as he was moribund and screaming and I did not want to wake the ward. I examined him. He had obvious gross bilateral cavitation and a severe pleural rub. I thought the latter was the cause of the pain and the screaming. I had

no morphia, just aspirin, which had no effect. I felt desperate. I knew very little Russian then and there was no one in the ward who did. I finally instinctively sat down on the bed and took him in my arms, and the screaming stopped almost at once. He died peacefully in my arms a few hours later. It was not the pleurisy that caused the screaming but loneliness. It was a wonderful education about the care of the dying. I was ashamed of my misdiagnosis and kept the story secret. (Wiffen, 2003)

These stories also recall the powerful visual image from the film 'Touching the void.' Jo, seriously wounded, crawls slowly and painfully along the icy mountain, expecting he will soon die. In a literally chilling scene he utters the cry of total human desolation and abandonment; yearning for human touch, he does not want to die alone. More than his desperate craving for food and water he longs for human embrace.

This cry of the human spirit is echoed every day in residential aged care facilities and in the broader community, for the research findings are unequivocal: loneliness, isolation, and boredom are the three plagues of our ageing society (Fratiglioni, Wang, Ericcson, Maytan, & Winblad, 2000; Mackenzie, 2000). One recent study has found that 97% of aged care residents lacked a sense of purpose that could be fulfilled through creative or spiritual activity (Fleming, 2004). Taking our cue from contemporary culture's emphasis on the individual as the sole arbiter of his or her life, the newly defined spirituality is directed inward, the symbols and rituals of a religious past are largely absent and faith's nourishing food scarcely available. This leaves older persons who are crying out for company, conversation, and touch, with nothing more tangible than an emphasis on their own privatised inner journey. It leaves those who yearn for signs of transcendent realities (prayer, worship, forgiveness) as sheep without a shepherd. This is not holistic care but spiritual fragmentation and religious reductionism. I am not suggesting that private contemplation and retreat to an 'inner world' are inconsequential in a person's spiritual journey. I *am* suggesting that if this is all we have to offer older people at the end of their lives then spirituality has become a mere fragment of our rather poor imagination.

CHRISTIANISING SPIRITUAL CARE

Christianity's task, (which has application for people of all faiths and no faith) is to answer the metaphysical questions: Who am I? To whom do I belong? Who will accompany me on life's journey and to whom may I be a companion? How can we, together, discover life's meaning at every stage of our created existence?

In a political world of broken promises, where we are urged to go confidently to the polls to vote on trust, we may well despair. In Christian theology, however, we make the outrageous claim that there is someone whom we can trust with our life and with our death; not because of some theoretical dogma, but because in the incarnation of the Son of God, Jesus Christ has lived our human life and died our human death. He had no private pathway to the Father whereby he could escape the loneliness and isolation in the garden where his closest friends had deserted him. He had no separate soul that could bypass the bodily torture, shame and ignominy of the cross. This was no private inner journey to find his own spirituality; this was a cosmic event for the salvation of the world. In the mystery of the cross and resurrection, Christianity lays claim to a full-bodied reality, manifest in the gift of Christ's own body, the flesh and blood that constitute the church. The resurrection claim is that we will be known, not in some vague, floating spiritual essence, but in our full-bodied humanity. While the mystery of cross and resurrection remains the subject of faith rather than sight, it is evident from Christian theology that the soul is not a separate entity, superior to the body. As Schmemann says:

> In essence, my body is my relationship to the world, to others; it is my life as communion and as mutual relationship. Without exception, everything in the body, in the human organism, is created for this relationship, for this communion, for this coming out of oneself.... [T]he body is not the darkness of the soul, but rather the body is its freedom, for the body is the soul as love, the soul as communion, the soul as life, the soul as movement. (Schmemann, 2003, pp. 42-43)

As embodied souls and ensouled bodies we are made for relationship, a communion of love that will not be thwarted, not even by death. Rather than fragile promises, we have in the life, death, resurrection, and ascension of Jesus Christ an eschatological hope, that is, not some vague otherworldly optimism, but the present reality of what is promised in the fulfillment of time.

The Language That's Missing

Spirituality's fragmentation–disembodied souls and soul-less bodies–is evident, as we have seen, in the problem-solving language of management. Fragmentation is also evident in the language that's missing. In a privatised, sanitised spirituality, there is no place for the sharing of wisdom, compassion, kindness, grace, love, faithfulness, mutuality, friendship, discernment, vulnerability, and partnership; not to mention joy and laughter, weeping, and sorrow. In the remaining space I would like to take up two of those 'forgotten' words: kindness and love.

In *An imaginary life*, David Malouf, the Australian writer, fictionalises the journey of the Roman poet Ovid who, in exile, encounters a wild boy, brought up among wolves in the snow. Gradually, the role of protector and protected are reversed as the two form a touching alliance. Ovid wrestles with the problem of befriending this boy, who is totally unattractive in every sense. How can he relate to this strange child with no language? Ovid says:

> I think and think. What must the steps be? How should I begin? Kindness, I know, is the way–and time. To reveal to him first what our kindness is, what our kind is; and then to convince him that we belong to the same kind. It is out of this that he must discover what he is. (Malouf, 1978, p. 77)

Ovid then asks what language will match this kindness.

> The language I am speaking of now, that I am almost speaking, is a language whose every syllable is a gesture of reconciliation. We knew that language once. I spoke it in my childhood. We must discover it again. (Malouf, 1978, p. 98)

The quintessential word that is absent from our professional language, even from most texts on spirituality, is *love*, the essence of human care, of which Jenson says:

> I am dependent for my humanity on yours. And that is a risky bet. There is not only risk here; there is mystery. For if I am dependent upon your humanity for mine, on whom are you dependent for yours? On me. . . . We wait endlessly for the word of love: each of us from the other, for none of us dares to speak it first. . . . And so I wait, and so do you, and the word of love is not spoken, to which our humanity would be the response. (Jenson, 1995, pp. 29-30)

CONCLUSION

To care for each person as an 'ensouled body' and 'embodied soul' is to acknowledge we are in the service of one another. For who of us is whole and in no need of healing? Who of us is capable of nurturing our own lives without the help of others, or without a transcendent Other?

In entering one another's stories, words like diagnose, define, and manage are replaced by trust, kindness, and love. Defined pathways and measurable outcomes are then replaced by risk, ambiguity, and mystery: the heart and soul and mind and body of human care.

REFERENCES

Anderson, R. S. (2003). *Spiritual caregiving as secular sacrament.* London and New York: Jessica Kingsley Publishers.

Baldacchino, D., & Draper, P. (2001). Spiritual coping strategies: A review of the nursing research literature. *Journal of Advanced Nursing, 34, 6,* 833-841.

Barth, K. (1960). *Church dogmatics, 11 1/2.* Edinburgh: T & T Clark.

Cobb, M. (2001). *The dying soul: Spiritual care at the end of life.* Buckingham: Open University Press.

Cobb, M., & Robshaw, V. (Eds.). (1998). *The spiritual challenge of health care.* Edinburgh: Churchill Livingstone.

Commonwealth of Australia. (2004). *Guidelines for a palliative approach in residential aged care.* Canberra: Edith Cowan University.

Cross, F. (Ed.). (1997). *The Oxford dictionary of the Christian church* (3rd ed.). Oxford: Oxford University Press.

Damasio, A. (1994). *Descartes' error: Emotion, reason, and the human brain.* New York: GP Putman's Sons.

Fleming, R. (2004). CPAT (Care Planning Assessment Tool)–Surprised by the obvious. *National Healthcare Journal, May,* 61.

Fratiglioni, L., Wang, H.-X., Ericcson, K., Maytan, M., & Winblad, B. (2000). Influence of social network on occurrence of dementia: A community-based longitudinal study. *The Lancet, 355 (April 15),* 1315-1319.

Goldsworthy, W. (2003). *Icons of grace: Ministry with the frail elderly.* Thornbury, Australia: Desbooks.

Hudson, R. (2003). Pastoral perspectives and policy issues in residential aged care. *Ministry, Society and Theology, 17, 1&2,* 10-31.

Hudson, R. (2004). Dementia and personhood: A living death or alive in God? *Colloquium: The Australian and New Zealand Theological Review, 36, 2,* 123-142.

Hudson, R., & Richmond, J. (2000). *Living, dying, caring: Life and death in a nursing home.* Melbourne: Ausmed Publications.

Jenson, R. W. (1995). *Essays in theology of culture.* Grand Rapids, MI: William B. Eerdmans Publishing Company.

Mackenzie, D. (2000). The Eden Alternative: A better way of life for residents and staff in aged care facilities. *National Healthcare Journal, (December)*, 21-23.

MacKinlay, E. (2004). The spiritual dimension of ageing. In A. Jewell (Ed.), *Ageing, spirituality and well-being*. 72-85. London and New York: Jessica Kingsley Publishers.

Malouf, D. (1978). *An imaginary life*. London: Chatto & Windus.

Orchard, H., & Clark, D. (2001). Tending the soul as well as the body: Spiritual care in nursing and residential homes. *International Journal of Palliative Nursing, 7, 11*, 541-546.

Palliative Care Australia. (2005). *Home page*. Retrieved 06.01.05, from the World Wide Web: *http://www.pallcare.org.au*

Pattison, S. (2001). Dumbing down the spirit. In H. Orchard (Ed.), *Spirituality in health care contexts*. 33-46. London and Philadelphia: Jessica Kingsley Publishers.

Picard, C. (1997). Embodied souls: The focus for nursing practice. *Journal of Holistic Nursing, 15, 3*, 41-53.

Rumbold, B. (Ed.). (2002). *Spirituality and palliative care*. Oxford: Oxford University Press.

Schmemann, A. (2003). *O death, where is thy sting?* (A. Vinogradov, Trans.). Crestwood, NY: St. Vladimir's Seminary Press.

Shamy, E. (2003). *A guide to the spiritual dimension of care for people with Alzheimer's disease and related dementia: More than body, brain and breath*. London: Jessica Kingsley Publishers.

Stumpf, S. E. (1994). *Philosophy: History & problems*. (5th ed.). New York: McGraw-Hill Inc.

Tarazi, P. N. (1999). *The New Testament: An introduction*. (Vol. 1 Paul and Mark). Crestwood, NY: St. Vladimir's Seminary Press.

Walter, T. (1997). The ideology and organization of spiritual care: Three approaches. *Palliative Medicine, 11*, 21-30.

Wiffen, P. (2003). The Cochrane collaboration: Pain, palliative, and supportive care. *Palliative Medicine, 17*, 75-77.

Spiritual Care:
Recognizing Spiritual Needs of Older Adults

Elizabeth MacKinlay, PhD, RN

SUMMARY. This paper explores aspects of spiritual needs and assessment, while emphasizing the importance of aged care providers being spiritually self-aware. The context of this exploration is meaning in life, spirituality and quality of life as experienced by older adults. Depression and dementia are frequently seen among older adults in residential aged care with resultant lowered quality of life. Pastoral and spiritual care may be used effectively to help alleviate depression and support older people who have dementia. However, to be able to provide appropriate spiritual care, spiritual needs should be assessed. Ways of assessing spiritual needs are suggested. *[Article copies available for a fee from The Haworth Document Delivery Service: 1-800-HAWORTH. E-mail address: <docdelivery@haworthpress.com> Website: <http://www.HaworthPress.com> © 2006 by The Haworth Press, Inc. All rights reserved.]*

KEYWORDS. Spirituality, spiritual needs, spiritual assessment, meaning in life, dementia, quality of life

Elizabeth MacKinlay, PhD, RN, is Director, Centre for Ageing and Pastoral Studies, and Associate Professor, School of Theology, Charles Sturt University, 15 Blackall Street Barton, ACT 2600, Australia (E-mail: emackinlay@csu.edu.au).

[Haworth co-indexing entry note]: "Spiritual Care: Recognizing Spiritual Needs of Older Adults." MacKinlay, Elizabeth. Co-published simultaneously in *Journal of Religion, Spirituality & Aging* (The Haworth Pastoral Press, an imprint of The Haworth Press, Inc.) Vol. 18, No. 2/3, 2006, pp. 59-71; and: *Aging, Spirituality and Palliative Care* (ed: Elizabeth MacKinlay) The Haworth Pastoral Press, an imprint of The Haworth Press, Inc., 2006, pp. 59-71. Single or multiple copies of this article are available for a fee from The Haworth Document Delivery Service [1-800-HAWORTH, 9:00 a.m. - 5:00 p.m. (EST). E-mail address: docdelivery@haworthpress.com].

SETTING A CONTEXT

"She's passed away" (people don't die), or "she's just attention seeking–she can't really be in pain"–said of a person with dementia. This was said, I must add, because her expressions of pain did not seem to be consistent with what the health care provider expected to see. Or the more general question: "Why can't they just be put out of their misery?"

These and other things are said around our nursing homes–these are not fiction, but statements from people working with older and frail nursing home residents. Those aged care workers are a reflection of the ignorance, myths, and ageist attitudes of our Western societies. Of course there are many workers in aged care who do not buy into the myths of ageing and dementia, many who give excellent care.

Too many older people in residential aged care are depressed. Levels of depression in high level care were found to range from 40-60% in a study of residents in Australian nursing homes (Fleming, 2001). Obviously, depression reduces quality of life for these residents. Facing ageism, depression, dementia, and one's own dying are some issues that are part of the nursing home experience.

I want to begin this paper with a quote from my friend Christine Bryden who has dementia; she is not in a nursing home yet, but she is struggling increasingly with cognition. I have been travelling with her as a companion on her journey into dementia, for most of the last decade. She has struggled through a lot of this time, with a question she first asked me back in about 1995: "Will I lose God as I travel into this disease?" Now, in 2005 in her second, and probably her last book, I have found her writing an inspirational part of this journey. I watch the struggle to know who she is emerging.

Christine has written:

> At the centre of our being lies the true self, what identifies us to be truly human, truly unique, and truly the person we were born to be. This is our spiritual heart, the centre from which we draw meaning in this rush from birth to death, whenever we pause long enough to look beyond our cognition, through our clouded emotions into what lies within. (Bryden, 2005 p. 163)

Christine is not old; she was diagnosed at age 47 with dementia (fronto-temporal), but now almost ten years later, she is very aware of the time of her life drawing in. She talks at times of how her daughters may respond to her if she is bed-bound, lying in a foetal position, and no longer able to communicate with them. Will they continue to come and visit? Will they try to communicate to her, when there is no sign of recognition from her? These are questions Christine and I have explored, yet not without hope. Her spiritual journey over this time has brought her to a time of strength and a deep sense of intimacy with God through Christ. She is not sitting back and waiting for death, but, rather, engaging with life to the full, as much as she is able and her energy levels allow.

These years of journeying with Christine as a spiritual guide have been a privileged time for me. I have learnt so much from her about what it is like to have dementia. She has challenged my nursing background and view of dementia, coming from a medical model, to see new possibilities in living with dementia and affirming these people in their individual journeys and struggle to find meaning in dementia.

What I have learned from Christine confirms the work of both Kitwood (1997) and Killick (2001), where they have raised issues of personhood and value of life of the person with dementia. Christine has been and is an inspiration to all who meet her. She is on a journey that she realizes will lead to death–we are partners on the road (Bryden, 2005).

There is a need to understand death in the context of life. Neither a view that focuses solely on life after death, with no regard to living life to the full, nor a view that focuses on 'live now' and denies the fact that we all will die will be sufficient. Mystery and the sacred intertwine in life and the process of dying. In this life, we often see "through a glass darkly." What does it mean when someone says, "I've still got life in me yet" when it seems they are so clearly facing pain and despair, and perhaps hopelessness, if we look at their situation on a rational basis.

We are tapping into the concept of spirituality–core meaning, deepest life meaning, and relationship; for many people this is worked out in relationship with God and others; for many others, there is no relationship with God, but relationship with others becomes primary. What lies at the centre, the heart of our being is from where we respond to all of life. Anger, hate, love, forgiveness, and hope come from the heart.

So often even now, when there seems to be a rising awareness of the spiritual in society, albeit, so often outside of mainstream religion, there has been little agreement on what is the spiritual domain; if everyone has it, if it ought to be addressed, and if so by whom, and how. At present, it seems there are more questions than answers.

Increasingly, within Australia, we are providing care within a multicultural and multifaith environment. Each of us associated with aged care needs first to be aware of our own spirituality and faith perspective, before we are able to meet the needs of others who may come from a different faith background.

WHO PROVIDES SPIRITUAL CARE?

Traditional Holders of the Spiritual Role: Chaplains and Other Clergy

Chaplains and pastoral carers have been seen as the traditional holders of the role of spiritual care. But now, in Western societies, there is a move for other professional groups to take on roles in spiritual care–nurses, doctors, social workers, diversional therapists, and others. These newcomers to spiritual care are still learning what the role entails; research and practice are moving together in emerging territory. I would suggest that even for clergy, the role may be extending as more research is conducted and findings incorporated into practice.

WHERE DO WE START IN SPIRITUAL CARE?

A great deal is beginning to appear in the literature of the different disciplines; from medical and psychosocial and nursing perspectives, the list of authors is rapidly growing longer (Atchley, 2000; Kimble and McFadden, 2003; Koenig, 1994; 1998; Koenig and Lawson, 2004; McFadden, Brennan, and Patrick, 2003; Moberg, 2001; Mowat and Ryan, 2003; Swinton, 2001).

Not all academics agree on the concept of spirituality, Draper and McSherry (2002) argue against the view that nurses should be "competent to assess the spiritual needs of patients. . . . " noting that this assumption is so widely accepted that it is expressed as a requirement for registration in the UK. Their position is that they cannot see evidence "that people share a common understanding of the existence of a spiritual realm" (p. 2). In response to this article, John Swinton (2002) notes the wealth of research that does provide evidence of the existence of spirituality, and its diversity, suggesting the need to explore how we might best develop this knowledge that will sensitise nurses and other health care workers to this dimension of care. What really is needed is confidence and education to enable effective practice.

It seems that if we are to recognise the spiritual dimension in health and ageing, to really make a difference for both ageing persons and older persons in need of care; the spiritual dimension can no longer be an optional extra to care; it is too important and too central to the well being of human beings. If we acknowledge the spiritual dimension as being equally a part of being human as is having a body and a mind, then we ought to address needs of the spirit with equal priority.

A number of people say to me: "I'm not really religious." When we talk about the spiritual dimension we are not only talking about religion–we are talking about spirituality, and religion is part of spirituality for a number of people (Figure 1).

FIGURE 1. Ways of Mediating the Spiritual Dimension

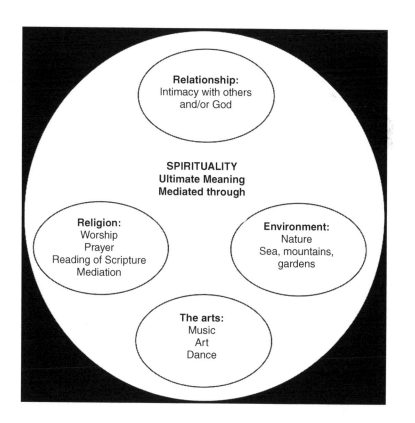

There are many definitions of spirituality; the one I am working with is:

> That which lies at the core of each person's being, an essential dimension which brings meaning to life. Constituted not only by religious practices, but understood more broadly, as relationship with God, however God or ultimate meaning is perceived by the person, and in relationship with other people. (MacKinlay, 2001a, p. 52)

This definition was developed out of PhD studies of independent living older people. The definition is a generic one that can be applied for people who have a religious faith and for those who have none. It also fits a humanistic framework, as it recognises that all humans have a spiritual dimension, and allows that people will live out their spiritual lives in various ways. This definition recognises the centrality of meaning for humans and, as well, the need for relationship with others.

It has in fact been said by a number of people that the 21st century will be the age of the spirit. Whether we mean a secular spirituality or a religious spirituality will vary greatly in different places and among different people. What will be important is that appropriate spiritual care is delivered wherever it is needed. This raises a critical question for care providers, and it is on this topic that I want to focus for the remainder of my paper. The topic is assessment of spiritual needs.

ASSESSING PSYCHOSOCIAL AND SPIRITUAL NEEDS

I believe there is a need to distinguish between these two dimensions. We use psychological tools to assess needs and well-being of the person's psychological status. For older people these range through the Mini Mental State Examination (MMSE), the Geriatric Depression Scale (GDS) and others. These instruments are not intentionally assessing the spiritual dimension, although the GDS does ask some questions that could be regarded as being of a spiritual nature. These instruments have been designed with different purposes in mind–the spiritual dimension is something else again. In fact, Hill and Pargament (2003) conclude their article *Advances in the conceptualization and measurement of religion and spirituality: Implications for physical and mental health research* with the words: "Already, there is evidence that religion and spirituality are distinctive dimensions that add unique explanatory power to the prediction of physical and mental health" (p. 74). That is, these dimensions may be different from other psychological and social constructs.

Likewise, we must ask, are we assessing needs or well-being? The concept of *well-being* is probably more useful for self-assessment of spiritual growth, or as an academic measure, than it is as a practical aide to assessment that will guide identification of spiritual needs. In my doctoral studies I used the Spiritual Health Inventory for Elderly (SHIE); this inventory was adapted from an assessment tool designed by a group of experts, but with no input from the target audience. On comparison with the factor analysis and the in-depth interviews from my research, the SHIE failed to predict sufficiently well to be accepted.[1] Essentially the SHIE did not take into account the importance of relationship for older people.

Assessing spiritual needs in a clinical setting should have one important aim–to assist in identifying the needs of the person for spiritual care.

BEING OPEN TO THOSE WE CARE FOR

We are attempting to tap into core meanings for individuals, to issues that lie at the very depth of their being. How can we tell what needs a frail elderly person has, or the needs of a person with dementia? How can we tell what psychosocial and spiritual needs they may have? Are we even sure of our own?

In fact, I believe that spiritual care is so important to quality of life and health, particularly in later life, and at any point when we face our own mortality, that the first prerequisite for effective spiritual care is that the person providing care is in touch with their own spirituality. So raising spiritual awareness among aged care staff is a crucial beginning to effective spiritual care. I have conducted workshops in aged care facilities on this topic (MacKinlay, 2001b).

WHOSE ROLE IS IT TO ASSESS SPIRITUAL NEEDS?

First, the resident may self-assess, after all this is very personal and we don't want to offend by asking (although we do ask if they have used their bowels).

Second, we could ask the resident. The resident would be the best authority on their spiritual being. However, it may be impossible for the resident to communicate their needs, such as following a stroke or sometimes in dementia. We may need to engage the assistance of family in the assessment.

Third, staff may assess, in this case certain assumptions are made by staff, based on their understanding of spirituality, and that may differ from how spirituality and spiritual needs are understood by the resident. Assumptions may include:

- That the person goes to church, therefore they have spiritual needs and these are met;
- Resident does not attend church services, therefore they have no spiritual needs; and
- The person has dementia–therefore they have no spiritual needs.

There are problems with these assumptions:

- The person may have moved to a new area and has no contacts with people who may provide for their spiritual needs;
- Not attending church does not mean that the person has no spiritual needs–if we consider that the spiritual dimension is part of being human, then there will be people who do not call themselves 'religious' and do not attend church, yet will acknowledge spiritual needs. Some may say these are existential needs; and
- People with dementia do have spiritual needs.

People with dementia do have spiritual needs; indeed, in later dementia this may be the main level of communication available; to cut them off from access to spiritual opportunities, e.g., rituals, liturgy music, is to cut off a life line to their souls.

Christine said: "As I travel towards the dissolution of my self, my personality, my very 'essence,' my relationship with God needs increasing support from you, my other in the body of Christ. Don't abandon me at any stage, for the Holy Spirit connects us. It links our souls, our spirits–not our minds or brains. I need you to minister to me, to sing with me, pray with me, to be my memory for me" (Bryden and MacKinlay, 2002, p. 74).

Thus assumptions staff make about the spiritual needs of residents may be wide of the mark.

What do we ask the resident? Perhaps it is important to first look at what we know of spirituality in later life; just what are we assessing?

WHAT DO WE ASK THE RESIDENT?

Perhaps it is important to first look at what we know of spirituality in later life, just what are we assessing? This model of spiritual tasks of ageing (MacKinlay, 2001a), Figure 2 was developed through my PhD and tested through further research since. In this model, meaning is at the centre of what it is to be human. Frail and older people, and those who are dying, may find God at the centre of their being, while others may find relationships with others providing central or core meaning in their lives (MacKinlay, 2001a).

Response to ultimate or core meaning may be through worship, art, music, dance, or nature and the environment. This response to meaning is a reaching out from our depth to otherness and to others. The spiritual tasks of ageing are dynamically inter-related, having core meaning at the centre. Tasks include finding final life meaning, transcending loss, finding new intimacy with God and/or others and finding hope, sometimes in the face of despair. Spiritual assessment must take account of all these factors, not only church attendance.

Elderly people will be at different places in their individual spiritual journeys. Some would not want to say they are on a spiritual journey at all, others would readily agree that the journey is spiritual (MacKinlay, 2001a). All would be able to respond to things of the spirit in some

FIGURE 2. Spiritual Tasks and Process of Ageing Spirituality in Later Life: Tasks–A Continuing Process

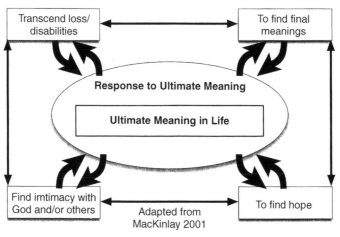

way–for instance, even without a faith or church background people are drawn to the beauty of art and music, to the beauty of a garden, trees, mountains, and the sea. There is something deep within the human soul that longs for these things. For many, symbols will connect them to others and to their God. For example–the liturgy of a church service that uses relevant symbols and rituals will facilitate connections with otherness.

Assessment of each of the spiritual tasks may provide indicators of need for growth and care. Care of the spirit should be intentional, and individualised, first identifying the spiritual needs of the person, so that these may be specifically addressed. Group work using pastoral care may also be useful. We are using this in current research on spiritual reminiscence with people who have dementia. Just to put a context on it, spirituality is both generic and specific; a broad undifferentiated spiritual or existential dimension may be the basis for the individual's life, or the spiritual dimension may be developed in specific ways, for instance, in the practice of a religion.

SO, HOW TO IDENTIFY NEEDS FOR SPIRITUAL CARE

There is a range of spiritual assessment tools available: some of these are based on assumptions from practice; some are based on anecdotal accounts of needs. Some attempt to quantify spirituality and use Likert scales to provide a score of spiritual well-being or spiritual need/distress or spiritual health.

When we work with the spiritual dimension, we are dealing with a different aspect of being human. Just as we developed psychological measures for assessing mental health and departures from it, so we need to develop spiritual measures that may be different again. I'm not sure that a score on spiritual well-being is going to be helpful to either the person whose score it is, or those who care for them.

I am suggesting two levels of assessment, based on my studies, mostly qualitative projects that have focused on finding important spiritual themes for older people–themes identified by the individuals themselves (MacKinlay, 2001a,b; MacKinlay, 2006).

First a Screening Assessment on Admission

This would be easy to use, not tiring to the resident or invasive, yet providing vital information on which to base care. It may be self-administered, be used by any staff, or may be family administered.

Second, an In-Depth Assessment Instrument

This may be used by pastoral carers or staff trained in spiritual or pastoral care. This would be done in the context of an interview, after admission to the aged care facility.

In this paper I have focused mainly on spiritual needs of people in residential aged care. I have outlined some assumptions underlying spiritual assessment and suggested a way towards developing assessment instruments.

There are three vital components here: staff, residents, and their families. Staff are still often reluctant to raise spiritual issues and to speak of dying and death with those they care for. We must acknowledge that the final career in life–moving towards death–is a real and important one. Giving permission for residents to speak openly about their fears, questions and concerns is an important beginning. Including families in the process as they feel able requires a sensitive yet open and supportive approach.

It may be that *all* who work with elderly people need to be comfortable with their own deeper values, concerns and beliefs–their sense of meaning and purpose in life, their hopes and fear, especially around dying, and their understanding of spirituality and faith. Recipients of care may be very sensitive to attitudes and comfort levels of staff in dealing with these issues.

CONCLUSION

Identification of spiritual needs is complex, but this does not mean it cannot be done, or that it should not be attempted. If we do not assess for spiritual needs, we will not even begin to notice these needs nor begin to find ways of addressing them. As I see it, spiritual needs underlie the psychosocial needs of people–they lie at the very core of what it is to be human. If we neglect these, especially for people at critical points of their lives and for those who are facing their frailty, dying, and death, then we neglect something equally important as failing to provide food and cleanliness to aged care residents. Spiritual care can no longer be an optional extra component of care.

Further guidelines for aged care accreditation need to be developed, and these guidelines may lie outside the scientific model. New understandings and new lenses are needed to develop appropriate assessments.

Yet, all of this is not going far enough; much that I have addressed in this paper is related to provision of spiritual care in residential aged care. Older people living independently also have spiritual needs, and rising levels of suicide among men over 85 years may be seen as a sign of a sense of hopelessness and lack of meaning and purpose in later life.

A healthy portfolio of spiritual strategies may well be protective against failure to thrive and depression in at least some older people–maybe this can be developed as part of the strategies to prevent social and spiritual isolation of older people living alone.

There is much to be done; we are in the early stages of the journey of discovery of the spiritual dimension in human beings in the 21st century.

NOTE

1. Factor analysis identified two factors (with an eigenvalue of more than 1) and these accounted for only 30.1 per cent of the variance of the SHIE (MacKinlay, 2001a, p. 41).

REFERENCES

Atchley, R. C. (2000). Spirituality. In T. R. Cole, R. Kastenbaum, & R. E. Ray, (Eds.), *Handbook of the humanities and aging.* 2d ed. New York: Springer, pp. 324-341.

Bryden, C. (2005). *Dancing with dementia: My story of living positively with dementia.* London: Jessica Kingsley Publishers.

Draper, P., & McSherry, W. (2002) A critical view of spirituality and spiritual assessment. *Journal of Advanced Nursing,* 39, 1, 1-2.

Folstein, M. F., Folstein, S. E., & McHugh, P. R. (1975). 'Mini-mental state': A practical method for grading cognitive state of patients for the clinician. *Journal of Psychiatric Research,* 12, 189-196.

Killick, J., & Allan, K. (2001). *Communication and the care of people with dementia.* Buckingham: Open University Press.

Killick, J. (2004). Dementia, identity, and spirituality. *Journal of Religious Gerontology,* 16, 3/4, 59-74.

Kimble, M. A., & McFadden, S. H. (Eds.). (2003). *Aging, spirituality and religion: A handbook, volume 2.* Minneapolis: Fortress Press.

Kitwood, T. (1997). *Dementia reconsidered.* Buckingham: Open University Press.

Koenig, H. G. (1994). *Aging and God: Spiritual pathways to mental health in midlife and later years.* New York: The Haworth Pastoral Press.

Koenig, H. G. (Ed.). (1998). *Handbook of religion and mental health.* San Diego: Academic Press.

Koenig, H. G., & Lawson, D. M. (2004). *Faith in the future: Healthcare, aging, and the role of religion.* Philadelphia: Templeton Foundation Press.

MacKinlay, E. B. (2001a). *The spiritual dimension of ageing.* London: Jessica Kingsley Publishers.

MacKinlay, E. B. (2001b). Understanding the ageing process: A developmental perspective of the psychosocial and spiritual dimensions. *Journal of Religious Gerontology*, 12, 3/4, 111-122.

MacKinlay, E. B. (2006). *Spiritual growth and care in the fourth age of life.* London: Jessica Kingsley Publishers.

McFadden, S. H., Brennan, M., & Patrick, J. H. (Eds.). (2003). *New directions in the study of late life religiousness and spirituality.* New York: The Haworth Pastoral Press.

Moberg, D. O. (Ed.). (2001). *Aging and spirituality: Spiritual dimensions of aging theory, research, practice, and policy.* New York: The Haworth Pastoral Press.

Mowat, H., & Ryan, D. (2003). Spiritual issues in health and social care: Practice into policy? *Journal of Religious Gerontology*, 14, 1, 51-68.

Swinton, J. (2001). *Spirituality and mental health care: Rediscovering a 'forgotten' dimension.* London: Jessica Kingsley Publishers.

Helping the Flame to Stay Bright: Celebrating the Spiritual in Dementia

John Killick, BA

SUMMARY. The medical model of dementia saw the organic nature of the condition as predominant. Recently the social model has come into prominence. This questions many of the prevailing assumptions about communication and awareness and offers a challenge to those in a caring role. Memory loss may have the effect of confining the person to present experience, but it may also give those without the condition the opportunity to appreciate qualities associated with being rather than doing. It opens up a positive approach to dementia, including the possible enhancement of creativity and spirituality. *[Article copies available for a fee from The Haworth Document Delivery Service: 1-800-HAWORTH. E-mail address: <docdelivery@haworthpress.com> Website: <http://www.HaworthPress. com> © 2006 by The Haworth Press, Inc. All rights reserved.]*

KEYWORDS. Communication, awareness, memory loss, personhood, challenge

John Killick, BA, is Associate Research Fellow, Dementia Services Development Centre, University of Stirling, Stirling, Scotland.

[Haworth co-indexing entry note]: "Helping the Flame to Stay Bright: Celebrating the Spiritual in Dementia." Killick, John. Co-published simultaneously in *Journal of Religion, Spirituality & Aging* (The Haworth Pastoral Press, an imprint of The Haworth Press, Inc.) Vol. 18, No. 2/3, 2006, pp. 73-78; and: *Aging, Spirituality and Palliative Care* (ed: Elizabeth MacKinlay) The Haworth Pastoral Press, an imprint of The Haworth Press, Inc., 2006, pp. 73-78. Single or multiple copies of this article are available for a fee from The Haworth Document Delivery Service [1-800-HAWORTH, 9:00 a.m. - 5:00 p.m. (EST). E-mail address: docdelivery@haworthpress.com].

Let us begin with a riddle. It comes from that amazing neurologist Oliver Sacks, and applies to more than dementia:

> A Who has a What–
> Will the What overcome the Who?
> Will the Who emerge through the What?
> Or will the two combine in a way
> that embraces and transcends the Condition?

(Sacks, 1996)

But I would like us to consider it specifically in the context of dementia, because of the threat which the condition poses to the personality. The first thing I ever published in the dementia field was a pamphlet entitled *Please Give Me Back My Personality!*, the title of which was an injunction from a lady with Alzheimer's who was painfully aware of the extent to which memory-loss inhibited her sense of coherence. The riddle is important because it encapsulates in its brief compass the whole history of attitudes to dementia up to the present. Until very recently the *What* dominated the field. The Medical Model held sway, the organic nature of dementia was uppermost, and few people gave the Who much credence as a surviving entity. Then along came a British psychologist Tom Kitwood amongst others to attempt to redress the balance. He insisted that the Who must take precedence over the *What*, and from this perspective proposed Personhood as the principle that should be given emphasis in all care. But the way he defined the concept was also important: "A standing or status which is bestowed on one human being, by others, in the context of relationship and social being. It implies recognition, respect and trust" (1997, p. 8). Now this is not a definition phrased in the context of medical concerns but taking full cognizance of social factors. It also downplays intellectual qualities in favour of a broader human spectrum. Individuals are to be valued for essential emotional and spiritual aspects of the personality. From this flows many of the positive aspects of dementia care which have been developed in the last decade or so.

One of the most remarkable developments lies in the number of personal accounts of dementia which have been published recently. Christine Boden, an Australian woman who combines strength of conviction with religious observance, and who is still in the early stages of the condition, posits what the future may hold for her in the following words: "The unique essence of 'me' is at my core, and this is what will remain with me at the end. I will be perhaps more truly 'me' than I have ever been" (1997, pp. 49-50).

An American woman, also with early dementia, has expressed similar sentiments in the following poem:

Burning Bright

Sometimes I picture myself
like a candle.
I used to be a candle about eight feet tall–
burning bright.
Now every day I lose
a little bit of me.
Someday the candle will be
very small.
But the flame will be
just as bright.

(Barb Noon, 2003)

One cannot underestimate the radical nature of these quotations. They (and similar passages from other authors) have an expressive power, and lead us to question many of the assumptions about communication and awareness which dominated the scene for so long. Although Barb Noon recognises that the candle will dwindle, she asserts that the spirit, represented by the flame, will be maintained and not lost in the general disintegration. Christine Boden even suggests that her self may be enhanced by the process to be undergone. It is as if the Alzheimer's, whilst destroying so much, actually has the capacity to hone the essential nature of the individual. Frena Gray Davidson, a professional carer in America, generalises about the process thus: "In many ways the deepest revelation of the Alzheimer journey is that it is a kind of passage from the mind into the heart" (1995, p. 7).

A more expansive explanation of what seems to be happening to people with dementia as it develops is offered by Tom Kitwood. He expresses it in the context of a description of an environment which is propitious for the maintenance of personhood:

> The ambience here is expansive and convivial. It is not simply a matter of special occasions, but any moment at which life is experienced as intrinsically joyful. Many people who have dementia,

despite their suffering, retain the capacity to celebrate. Celebration is the form of interaction in which the division between caregiver and cared-for comes nearest to vanishing completely. The ordinary boundaries of ego have become diffuse, and selfhood has expanded. In some mystical traditions, this is the meaning of spirituality. (Kitwood, 1997, pp. 90-91)

And in another quotation he makes an important distinction between the mind-set of the caregiver and the psyche of the person with the condition, which may, unless adaptation is possible, lead to dissonance:

Contact with dementia or other forms of severe cognitive disability should take us out of our customary patterns of over-busyness, hypercognitivism and extreme talkativity into a way of being in which emotion and feeling are given a much larger place. People who have dementia, for whom the life of the emotions is often intense, and without the ordinary forms of inhibition, may have something important to teach the rest of humankind. (Kitwood, 1997, p. 5)

Of course acknowledging insight and sensitivity as essential qualities found in many people with dementia poses a challenge to those who would care for them. Some may question whether they are up to meeting that challenge. It requires us to look into ourselves for our own personal resources, and to expend them quite freely and intensely. The rewards, as Kitwood indicates, may be rich, but not without considerable risk-taking on our part.

Another aspect of communicating with and valuing the experience of people with dementia is the need to appreciate the different time-scale within which they may be seen to operate. Memory-loss may have the effect of confining the person largely to present experience, with little awareness of past or future. It may be difficult for those without dementia to adapt to a now-oriented existence. Our whole life-strategy is geared to awareness of change and planning for a possible future. Debbie Everett, a hospital chaplain in Canada, provides a pair of metaphors which encapsulate this memorably:

For those of us who are cognitively intact time is like a stream of water in which we float with the current. For someone with Alzheimer's Disease time is frozen into individual snowflakes which touch the skin and melt. (Everett, 1996, p. 85)

This is yet another area in which the person with dementia may have much to teach us. Marie de Hennezel, a French psychologist, shows us what we have to gain: "We need to savour every moment of being alive. To know when to stand still and listen to the soft rustling of existence" (1997, p. 100).

I return to the carer and the challenge we face in accompanying another person on their voyage into the unknown which is dementia. It is not wrong to feel faint-hearted at contemplating the days and months ahead. It is not wrong to be afraid of what lies in the future. It is not wrong to feel powerless in a situation where the obstacles may seem too many and too high. But the truth is we will be unable to function in this situation if we allow faint-heartedness, fear, and powerlessness to dominate our attempts to remain alongside and reassure the person with the condition.

Debbie Everett puts these issues in the following way:

> We must not fear the unknown, or the insufficiency or powerlessness we feel when we are with someone with dementia. Yes, we can experience it but we must not allow the fear to keep us away. The powerlessness that may occur when caring for a person with dementia has a lot to do with the caregiver's inability to value other means of communication than just words. This fear multiplies the feeling of meaninglessness about ministering to these people. When we see only meaninglessness, commitment is often lost. Surrender to the mystery of the future means admitting the possibility of suffering. Real care for those affected by dementia only takes place when the walls of fear have been removed. (Everett, 1996, p. 42)

We concentrate necessarily on the personhood of the one with dementia, as that is so difficult to maintain in all circumstances. But we should be placing equal emphasis on the individuality of the carer in whatever context. Communication requires selflessness and a daring which takes its toll over time, and resources need regular replenishment. We are none of us physically or spiritually inexhaustible, and support and respite are essential parts of the equation if the flame is to be recognised and cherished.

Marie de Hennezel reminds us that it is possible, once such safeguards are in place, for the act of giving to be self-renewing:

One actually is less exhausted by a total involvement of self–provided one knows how to replenish one's reserves–than by the attempt to barricade oneself behind one's defences. I have often seen for myself how the medical personnel who protect themselves the most are also those who complain the most of being exhausted. Those who give themselves, however, also recharge themselves at the same time. (De Hennezel, 1997, p. 130)

Given this perspective, dementia offers one of the great challenges of our time. If we fail to meet it our spirituality and our resolve will have been found wanting. If we take it on, it is no exaggeration to say that it has the potential for enhancing our whole conception of what it is to be human.

REFERENCES

Boden, C. (1997). *Who shall I be when I die?* London: Harper Collins.

Davidson, F. G. (1995). *Alzheimer's: A practical guide for carers.* London: Piatkus.

De Hennezel, M. (1997). *Intimate death: How the dying teach us to live.* New York: Little Brown.

Everett, D. (1996). *Forget-me-not: The spiritual care of people with Alzheimer's.* Edmonton, Canada: Inkwell Press.

Kitwood, T. (1997). *Dementia reconsidered.* Buckingham: Open University Press.

Noon, B. (2003). In S. Benson & J. Killick (Eds.), *Creativity in dementia care calendar 2004.* Hawker: London.

Sacks, O. (1996). Quotation authorized by the writer.

"I Am Just an Ordinary Person . . .":
Spiritual Reminiscence in Older People
with Memory Loss

Corinne Trevitt, RN, MN, Grad Dip Gerontics
Elizabeth MacKinlay, PhD, RN

SUMMARY. One of the greatest challenges to people diagnosed with dementia is their search for meaning leading to the development of effective coping strategies as their memory loss and confusion progresses. The challenge for carers is to learn ways of entering the world of people who have difficulties communicating and have behaviour problems, as-

Corinne Trevitt, RN, MN, Grad Dip Gerontics, is Academic Associate, Centre for Ageing and Pastoral Studies, Charles Sturt University, 15 Blackall Street, Barton, ACT, Australia (E-mail: ctrevitt@csu.edu.au).

Elizabeth MacKinlay, PhD, RN, is Director, Centre for Ageing and Pastoral Studies, and Associate Professor, School of Theology, Charles Sturt University, 15 Blackall Street, Barton, ACT, Australia.

This paper presents results from the following research projects: MacKinlay, Trevitt, & Hobart (2002), *The search for meaning: Quality of life for the person with dementia*, funded by University of Canberra Collaborative Research Grant. MacKinlay, Trevitt, & Coady (2002-05). *Finding meaning in the experience of dementia: The place of spiritual reminiscence work*, funded by an Australian Research Council (ARC) Linkage Grant LP0214980.

[Haworth co-indexing entry note]: " 'I Am Just an Ordinary Person . . .' : Spiritual Reminiscence in Older People with Memory Loss." Trevitt, Corinne, and Elizabeth MacKinlay. Co-published simultaneously in *Journal of Religion, Spirituality & Aging* (The Haworth Pastoral Press, an imprint of The Haworth Press, Inc.) Vol. 18, No. 2/3, 2006, pp. 79-91; and: *Aging, Spirituality and Palliative Care* (ed: Elizabeth MacKinlay) The Haworth Pastoral Press, an imprint of The Haworth Press, Inc., 2006, pp. 79-91. Single or multiple copies of this article are available for a fee from The Haworth Document Delivery Service [1-800-HAWORTH, 9:00 a.m. - 5:00 p.m. (EST). E-mail address: docdelivery@haworthpress.com].

sisting them to communicate more effectively by responding to their interests and needs, and listening to their emotions expressed in various ways. Strategies are being developed for supporting and affirming personhood in those people who are often isolated and withdrawn from even their closest friends and relatives. Spiritual reminiscence work is one way of helping older people with memory loss find meaning in their lives as they cope with the day to day difficulties of memory loss and prepare for death.

This paper will present the results from indepth interviews from 16 participants in a larger study exploring memory loss and spiritual reminiscence. Themes arising from the data analysis revolve around notions of relationships, loneliness, family and attendance at worship. *[Article copies available for a fee from The Haworth Document Delivery Service: 1-800-HAWORTH. E-mail address: <docdelivery@haworthpress.com> Website: <http://www.HaworthPress.com> © 2006 by The Haworth Press, Inc. All rights reserved.]*

KEYWORDS. Dementia, memory loss, spiritual reminiscence work, communication, meaning in life

INTRODUCTION

In 2002, we began a study that was designed to give those with dementia a voice to describe their lives by talking about hopes, fears, and the ways they sought meaning in their lives (MacKinlay, Trevitt, & Coady, 2002-2005). There have been a number of studies examining the effects of dementia on families and friends but few studies ask questions and listen to the person with dementia. We used spiritual reminiscence work (Gibson, 1998, 2004) to study the experience of dementia and the spiritual dimension, focussing on how people with dementia find meaning and develop coping strategies. This was a collaborative project between Charles Sturt University and three industry partners: Anglican Retirement Community Services, Wesley Gardens Aged Care, and Mirinjani Village Aged Care.

This paper will present the results from indepth interviews from 16 participants from the study and explores memory loss and spiritual reminiscence. Early themes arising from the data analysis revolve around notions of relationships, loneliness, family, and attendance at worship.

This paper will also briefly discuss some of the interactions observed during the spiritual reminiscence sessions.

BACKGROUND

Dementia is a significant issue in an ageing society. Dementia prevalence is expected to double every 5.1 years after age 65, affecting 24% of those over the age of 85 (Henderson & Jorm, 1998). In residential aged-care facilities only 20% of residents are identified as not having dementia (AIHW, 2004). Dementia is responsible for progressive cognitive and functional impairment over a period of years, with great cost to individuals, families and the community. Management of the condition is both costly and complex, with a current focus on maintaining those affected at home for as long as possible. For most, institutional care is required during the later stages. Admission to aged-care facilities usually occurs as a result of unmanageable behaviour such as aggression, incontinence, or being unable to be left living alone for a range of safety issues.

While there is continuing research into both the causes of dementia and pharmacological cures, the greatest need presently is to find ways to enhance quality of life for those diagnosed with dementia. This means there needs to be an emphasis on understanding the world of the person with dementia; on communication that can tap into the 'inner core of being' of the person with dementia; and thoughtful strategies to manage the most disturbing behavioural challenges in a setting that is caring, secure, and meaningful.

In recent years the power of reminiscence work, that is, the ability to review one's life and its meaning, has been recognised as:

> part of a natural healing process and it represents one of the underlying human capacities on which psychotherapy depends. The life review should be recognised as a necessary and healthy process in daily life as well as a useful tool in the mental health care of older people. (Butler, 1995, xviii)

For the person who has dementia, this normal process of meaning-making becomes complicated, and may be blocked. This does not mean that people who have dementia can no longer find and/or respond to meaning, but that we may need to find ways to reach and support them in their increasing confusion and communication difficulties, as they seek to find meaning in the experience of dementia.

There have been a number of different types of reminiscence identified. Gibson (1998) discusses the use of reminiscence with people who have dementia, particularly focusing on issues of personhood and quality of life. Gibson carefully distinguishes between 'general' and 'specific' reminiscence in working with people who have dementia. Her work was conducted with people who have severe dementia and she found that 'specific' work was more effective for these people, and easier to do on a one-to-one basis. The term general reminiscence covers "well-prepared work that uses a variety of multi-sensory triggers to stimulate shared conversation on an agreed topic or theme which relates loosely to the known background and interests of the participants." Specific reminiscence consisted of "carefully selected, highly focused, concentrated consistent efforts to stimulate recall and conversation using carefully selected triggers known to closely approximate the detailed life-history of the participant" (Gibson, 1998, p. 16).

Spiritual reminiscence is a particular way of communicating with older people. Rather than general reminiscence when a life story may be discussed, spiritual reminiscence asks questions about meaning in life, joy, sadness, grief, and regrets. Within spiritual reminiscence we speak of hopes and fears for the future, what people want from the last years of their lives, who they can share deep concerns with and whether they feel that their spiritual needs are being met. We ask questions about a person's relationship with God or other deity, whether they pray, meditate, or engage in other spiritual practices.

THE STUDY

One hundred and thirteen older adults resident in aged-care facilities, all of whom had a medical diagnosis of dementia, participated in the study. The study had ethical clearance from the university and each of the aged-care facilities. Consent was gained from each of the participants and their relatives/guardians. After consent was obtained, demographic data was collected and each participant took part in an indepth interview. These participants were then allocated to spiritual reminiscence groups to participate in small group work over a period of either six weeks or six months. In these small groups (three to six participants), a facilitator (a member of facility staff–a diversional therapist, pastoral carer, or chaplain) would lead a discussion focused on spiritual reminiscence.

There Were Four Approaches Used for Data Collection

1. Prior to the beginning of the spiritual reminiscence groups each participant had: an indepth interview and collection of demographic data; completion of the Bird Dementia Scale; and Mini Mental State Exam (MMSE) (Folstein et al., 1975).
2. A facilitator would lead a discussion on spiritual reminiscence in small groups for either six weeks or six months. All groups were tape recorded. An observer (research assistant) noted all non-verbal interactions in the groups.
3. A behaviour rating scale (INTERACT) was completed on all participants before and after each small group by the research assistant.
4. Staff focus groups were held following the project to allow them to describe their observations of behaviour change in the participants.

Questions that guided the indepth interviews and the reminiscence groups were aimed to encourage participants to share their memories and describe what gave them meaning in their lives. The following are examples of questions asked:

- Looking back over your life what do you remember with joy? With sadness?
- Tell me about the emotional and spiritual supports you have. Are these from family, friends?
- What things do you worry about?
- What gives meaning to your life?
- What are the good things in your life?
- Do you have any fears?
- What are the hardest things in your life just now?
- Do you have an image of God? What is this image like?
- As you get to the end of your life, what do you look forward to?

Data analysis was undertaken using QSR N6–a computer based qualitative data analysis package that helps the researcher to identify themes in the data. Both researchers code and then check each other's coding to ensure rigor of the emerging themes.

For this paper we have randomly identified 16 indepth interviews to report. At this stage of the project we are still in the early stages of data analysis. Early themes arising from the data analysis revolve around notions of relationships, loneliness, family, and attendance at worship and how these combine to give a sense of purpose, humour and insight into their illness and living circumstances.

RESULTS

As we read the transcripts of interviews we are frequently struck by the capacity of these people with dementia. The participants in this project are not newly diagnosed–in fact they have progressed to the stage where they require at least low level residential aged care and in some cases high level care. A number of participants could not understand why we were interested in their life story. Many of them professed not having anything to tell: "I'm just an ordinary person. . . . " reflects this response. The themes that emerged from this data were concerned with relationship, meaning, worship, insight, and humour.

Relationship and Meaning

Relationship was a very important part of the lives of our participants. When asked about meaning in life, most responded that the love and support of their families was the most important part of their lives. Many spoke of the loss of their parents and siblings as continuing to have a significant effect on them. The importance of the remembrance of relationship after the death of a loved one is supported by de Vries (2001). Where it was once thought that successful grieving led to the closure of the relationship with the deceased, it is now suggested that grief work includes resolution of the relationship to a continuing but different place in the surviving person's life. Thus the vivid and continuing effects of the lost relationships of these people with dementia are typical of an expected outcome of grief, even though the person with dementia may at times not be able to identify the particular nature of the lost relationship. A number of the participants speak of loneliness and loss of friends:

I am alone more.

I don't have many people now. I had some very nice people you know when I was younger, and they were best friends. I don't have a friend now.

It would be nice to have someone to talk to.

It is interesting to note that although each of these people lives in an aged care facility, they describe being alone and not having anyone to talk to. This was also found among aged care residents who were cognitively intact (MacKinlay, 2001b); however, the importance of relationship for people who have dementia is not always recognized.

For a number of respondents the absence of their family was the hardest thing in their life just now:

> *. . . not having my family around me*

For another, her greatest regret was not having her spouse with her:

> *. . . not being home with my husband*

Other participants however, found meaning in their activities:

> *Oh just walking*

> *To keep healthy, mix with people, go to bed and sleep peacefully*

> *To have a tidy workspace*

Others find their God and church add meaning.

> *. . . as I live a life well pleasing the Lord*

Still others had a different approach. For one meaning was in the routine of daily life:

> *. . . food and sleep*

Yet another participant was more pragmatic

> *I'm over meaning*

Worship

The majority of participants in this group either attended or used to attend church. Many of them continue to pray either on their own or in an organized group. They have very vivid early memories of church and God.

> *My mother told me about God when I was about 4 (years old)*

> *I used to go to Sunday School*

One of the questions asked was whether they had any fears; most said they had none.

> *No can't say, I trust in the Lord*

> *No I don't think so. . . . people have been kind to me . . .*

> *No . . . I don't let fears rule my life*

In a similar study of spirituality with a group of cognitively intact older people living independently, their greatest fear was of developing dementia (MacKinlay, 2001a). While it might be argued that those with dementia were unaware of whether they had fears, their conversation on this topic would suggest that these people with dementia had come to a place of acceptance of their situations. However, it is also suggested that fears and apprehension may be present in people who have dementia, particularly in the earlier stages of dementia, or later, if they have not been able to deal effectively with their diagnosis and finding meaning in the experience of dementia.

Insight

It is often assumed that those with dementia have reduced or no insight into their situation. Participants in this study seemed to be able to speak and share significant issues of life and death. They also expressed a satisfaction with their lives and an acceptance of death. When asked what they look forward to now as they approach the end of their lives, there were a variety of positive responses. It is interesting to note that frequently we feel uncomfortable about asking questions related to dying and death, but these participants not only welcomed the questions but were able to describe their hopes. This seems to oppose the idea of lack of insight.

Well, I am ready to go. I have lived my life

I just take each day as it comes . . . if it doesn't come, well that's it. . . .

I know I am going to die, everybody will die

I look forward to going to heaven

Humour

Humor was evident in many of the answers–there was frequently laughter during the interviews. Many responses were not only amusing, but again demonstrated some ability to of these people to recognize their situation. One interchange during an interview illustrates an example of the participant recognizing and correcting their mistake and then having a good laugh over it.

> *Participant: Well you are lovely and young and very lucky, cause I am 89. I was born in 1818 I think.*
>
> *Interviewer: 1918?*
>
> *Participant: 1918? Oh! (lots of laughter).*

Or admission of loss of memory:

> *A lot of us have got short term memory, we can tell you what happened 60 years ago.*
>
> *I have got the most dreadful short-term memory, short term. It's most embarrassing sometimes (laughter)*

In another interview one of the participants finishes up with

> *don't blame other people when you can blame yourself*

DISCUSSION

There has been much discussion in the literature about the capacity of those with dementia to communicate and comprehend the reality of their lives, or even to recognize others (Bornat, 1994; Keck, 1996; Simpson & Simpson, 1999; Kitwood, 1997). Many relatives talk about how the person they knew is 'gone,' about how there is no point in visiting regularly because there is no memory of these visits. Frequently a family member will speak of being distressed when their relative fails to remember a recent outing. Christine Boden, a woman living with dementia, made a plea for us not to stop taking her for a walk when she can no longer remember it, emphasizing the importance of the moment of the experience (Boden, 1998). In her later book Christine notes that she is more and more conscious of only the moment, but that moment is still important (Bryden, 2005). Relatives may say things like: "I can't face visiting anymore. I can't bear to see him like this"; "This is a living death"; or "Shoot me if I ever get like that" (Hudson, 2004, p. 212). Hudson (2004) identifies the three dreaded "D"s–death, dying, and dementia and how these are seen as pessimistic for staff, relatives, and the older person. Often the process of dementia is coloured by the difficulties of communication and associated fear that prevent any real connection between the person with dementia and others.

However, when we examined the interactions in the interviews with these people, their memories of happy and sad times are very clear. They also speak lovingly of their family–making excuses for why family members cannot visit as often as they would like them to. They grieve over losses of parents decades ago. Each of the participants was able to talk about what they hoped from the remainder of their lives. All the interviewees in this paper declared that they were ready for death. Many appreciated the fact that they still had their health and felt they had experienced full lives.

McFadden (2003) writes that by observing the everyday actions of people living with dementia you can see that hope is not destroyed by the disease. In fact, watching the interactions within these groups, it is evident there is a vitality that is sometimes not witnessed in the usual environment of an aged care facility. The task for carers is to nurture and encourage the type of environment that allows these people to interact in such a meaningful way.

From the responses and the interactions in these interviews we might argue that although the respondents have dementia they are experiencing transcendence. They describe their lives as full, valuable, and worth living. Although Erikson was reporting the findings of octogenarians who were cognitively intact, he found that many of them found life full, valuable and worth living (Erikson, 1986). Can it not be the same for those who live with dementia?

Palliative care for those with dementia needs to address issues of spirituality as well as issues of physical comfort and psychosocial well being. Hudson (2004, p. 213) describes this palliative care as having a focus on the "particular meaning of this particular experience for this particular resident at this particular time in his or her unique family context." Spiritual reminiscence is a way of meeting the person in this particular way. By asking questions about the person's hopes and fears, joys and sadness, and the meaning in their lives, we are offering a particular experience and meeting with the person on an individual level. Carers may feel inadequate asking these types of questions–but the risk is worth it–offering yourself and being willing to listen is particularly rewarding for those in aged care and invaluable for residents.

Although this paper based on 16 indepth interviews, we would like to share some of the observations of the groups that met weekly to discuss issues of spiritual reminiscence. The research assistants helped prepare for each weekly session and kept a journal of non-verbal behaviours and environment factors during the group sessions, as well as tape recording the groups and completing behaviour ratings of the participants before and after each weekly meeting. The following observations are from the weekly journals. There is a lot of humour in the interactions–and evidence of much caring between participants. The research assistant observing and journaling interactions, describes how one participant holds the hand of another as she talks about a sad occasion. In one interaction between participants there is obviously the opportunity for ambiguity. The participant not only recognizes this, but corrects it.

In two of the six month groups, a group member died before the end of the period of group sessions. The remaining group members engaged in grief work, acknowledging and discussing the death and loss of the person from the group. This is frequently very difficult to do in aged-care facilities, as places are filled with new residents. In one of the groups, the husband of one of the group members died during the period of the group meeting. At the end of the six months of group meetings she said how much comfort she had received from the group. They offered her a level of social support that is usually unavailable in aged care.

In another group, the diversional therapist has noted that one of the participants is much more animated and ready to join in than she has ever seen before. Participants remember the meeting days and times for the small groups and are ready to form the group prior to the meeting time, even though they may forget and need prompting for most other activities. It is noted that this is not the 'norm' for activities in the aged care facility. On completion of the groups, some of the participants have been noted to be animatedly chatting as they go to the dining room. However, once separated from the other reminiscence group members they attempt to engage the people on each side of them at dinner, but soon give up as they receive no response. Again, they become listless, quiet and uninterested in what is going on around them. On the conclusion of one group meeting a participant said 'thank you for this. We do not get to talk about these things usually.'

What is it about the spiritual reminiscence group that encourages this positive interaction? One suggestion is that the participants are interacting in a safe and comfortable environment. The facilitator ensures that the focus and control in the group sessions is lightly held, that the group members are affirmed and free to interact with others in the group. Over a period of some weeks, the group members get to know each other, and may begin to form new friendships. Further analysis of the data from this large qualitative study is still to be completed.

CONCLUSION

The journey into death is life's final career (Heinz, 1994; MacKinlay, 2001a). An important task in the final career is to make sense of the life we have lived, to find meaning in the whole of the journey. This task of finding meaning may be complicated by the onset of dementia, making it harder for the person to work through the process of finding meaning. Spiritual reminiscence is a way of exploring and finding final life meanings. This may be a valuable strategy for assisting people with dementia to cope with the experience of dementia and to transcend their losses and come to acceptance of their lives. Spiritual reminiscence is thus a way of providing a preparation for the final career and a lead into palliative care to those with dementia.

The interviews have given us as researchers a very special insight into the lives of this group of older people living with memory loss. Carers and relatives are in a unique position to interact in this privileged and personal way, in the process of spiritual reminiscence, walking the journey into the meaning of dementia.

REFERENCES

Australian Institute of Health and Welfare. (2004). *The impact of dementia on the health and aged care system.* AIHW Cat. No AGE 37. Canberra: AIHW.

Boden, C. (1998). *Who will I be when I die?* Pymble: Harper Collins Religious.

Bornat, J. (Ed.) (1994). *Reminiscence reviewed.* Buckingham: Open University Press.

Bryden, C. (2005). *Dancing with dementia: My story of living positively with dementia.* London: Jessica Kingsley Publishers. 135.

Butler, R. N. (1995). Forward. In B. K. Haight, & J. D. Webster. (Eds.), *The art and science of reminiscence: Theory, research, methods, and applications.* Washington, DC: Taylor and Francis.

De Vries, B. (2001). Grief: Intimacy's reflection. *Generations,* Summer, 75-80.

Erikson, E. H., Erikson, J. M., & Kivnick, H. Q. (1986). *Vital involvement in old age.* New York: W. W. Norton & Co.

Folstein, M. F., Folstein, S. E., & McHugh, P. R. (1975). Mini-mental state: A practical method for grading cognitive state of patients for the clinician. *Journal of Psychiatric Research,* 12, 189-196.

Gibson, F. (1998). *Reminiscence and recall: A guide to good practice.* London: Age Concern Books.

Gibson, F. (2004). *The past in the present: Using reminiscence in health and social care.* Baltimore: Health Professions Press.

Haight, B. K., & Webster, J. D. (Eds.) (1995). *The art and science of reminiscence: Theory, research, methods, and applications.* Washington, DC: Taylor and Francis.

Henderson, A., & Jorm, A. (1998). *Dementia in Australia. Aged and community care service development and evaluation report.* No. 35. Canberra: AGPS.

Heinz, D. (1994). Finishing the story: Aging, spirituality and the work of culture. *Journal of Religious Gerontology,* 9, 1, 3-19.

Hudson, R. (Ed.) (2003). *Dementia nursing: A guide to practice.* Melbourne: Ausmed Publications.

Hudson, R. (2003). Palliative care. In R. Hudson, (Ed.), *Dementia nursing: A guide to practice.* Melbourne: Ausmed.

Keck, D. (1996). *Forgetting whose we are: Alzheimer's disease and the love of God.* Nashville, TN: Abington.

Kitwood, T. (1997). *Dementia reconsidered.* Buckingham: Open University Press.

MacKinlay E. B. (2001a). *The spiritual dimension of ageing.* London: Jessica Kingsley Publishers.

MacKinlay E. B. (2001b). Health, healing and wholeness in frail elderly people. *Journal of Religious Gerontology,* 13, 2, 25-34.

MacKinlay, E. B., Trevitt, C., & Hobart, S. (2002). *The search for meaning: Quality of life for the person with dementia.* University of Canberra Collaborative Grant 2001. Unpublished Project Report, February 2002.

MacKinlay, E. B., Trevitt, C., & Coady, M. (2002-2005). *Finding meaning in the experience of dementia: The place of spiritual reminiscence work.* Australian Research Council. Linkage Grant.

Who Is Afraid of Death?
Religiousness, Spirituality,
and Death Anxiety in Late Adulthood

Paul Wink, PhD

SUMMARY. Data from a sample of predominantly white, Christian men and women born in Northern California in the 1920s ($N = 155$) were used to test the hypothesis that traditional, church-centered religiousness and de-institutionalized spiritual seeking exemplify distinct, but equally adaptive, ways of approaching fear of death in old age. Although both religiousness and spirituality were related to positive psychosocial functioning (an integrated identity and involvement in everyday activities), only religiousness served as a buffer against the fear of death. This effect was consistent with the greater emphasis on conventionality and acceptance of social norms that characterized individuals high in religiousness. The absence of a relation between spirituality and fear of death reflected the spiritual individual's emphasis on personal searching, cre-

---

Paul Wink, PhD, is affiliated with the Department of Psychology, Wellesley College, Wellesley, MA 02482 USA (E-mail: pwink@wellesley.edu).

The author would like to thank Michele Dillon for her helpful comments.

The data for this study were collected with a grant from the Open Society Institute awarded to Paul Wink. This research was funded by grant #10406 from the John Templeton Foundation awarded to Paul Wink and Michele Dillon.

[Haworth co-indexing entry note]: "Who Is Afraid of Death? Religiousness, Spirituality, and Death Anxiety in Late Adulthood." Wink, Paul. Co-published simultaneously in *Journal of Religion, Spirituality & Aging* (The Haworth Pastoral Press, an imprint of The Haworth Press, Inc.) Vol. 18, No. 2/3, 2006, pp. 93-110; and: *Aging, Spirituality and Palliative Care* (ed: Elizabeth MacKinlay) The Haworth Pastoral Press, an imprint of The Haworth Press, Inc., 2006, pp. 93-110. Single or multiple copies of this article are available for a fee from The Haworth Document Delivery Service [1-800-HAWORTH, 9:00 a.m. - 5:00 p.m. (EST). E-mail address: docdelivery@haworthpress.com].

doi:10.1300/J078v18n02_08

ativity, and the positive use of reminiscence. The implications of the findings for the management of death anxiety in old age are discussed. *[Article copies available for a fee from The Haworth Document Delivery Service: 1-800-HAWORTH. E-mail address: <docdelivery@haworthpress.com> Website: <http://www.HaworthPress.com> © 2006 by The Haworth Press, Inc. All rights reserved.]*

KEYWORDS. Death anxiety, religiousness, spirituality, psychosocial functioning, aging

Death anxiety is portrayed in negative terms as a sign of lack of self-realization (e.g., Wong, 2000) and in a positive light as evidence of sufficient ego-strength and personal openness in confronting the most fundamental human experience (e.g., Becker, 1973). These two views are typically presented as offering alternative rather than complementary views of the relation between fear of death and positive psychosocial functioning. This study investigated the relation among religiousness, spirituality, and fear of death to test the hypothesis that there are two distinct, yet equally adaptive, ways of approaching death anxiety in old age.

DEATH ANXIETY
AND POSITIVE PSYCHOSOCIAL FUNCTIONING

The more commonly accepted view of death anxiety states that fear of death is a sign of lack of fulfillment or self-realization that leads to regret and despair (e.g., Erikson, 1963; Wong, Reker, & Gesser, 1994; Yalom, 1980). On this view, a healthy developmental sequence leads from a basic sense of trust in childhood to self-realization in adulthood, followed by the attainment of ego integrity that allows the older adult to accept death with equanimity (Erikson, 1963). In other words, a "healthy view" of death anxiety (Firestone, 1994) is based on the premise that individuals are not so much afraid of death as of an incompleteness in their lives or the lack of self-fulfillment (Goodman, 1981). As stated by Kubler-Ross (1997), "Dying is nothing to fear . . . it all depends on how you have lived" (p. 286). Empirical support for the "healthy view" is provided by numerous studies showing a negative relation between death anxiety and self-acceptance and life satisfaction (e.g., Loretto & Templer, 1986; Neimeyer & van Brunt, 1995; Tomer & Eliason, 2000).

An alternative, "morbid" view (Firestone, 1994) of the relation between fear of death and psychosocial functioning assumes that death anxiety is a given of human existence because we are the only species to realize our mortality, an insight that contributes to the dread of non-existence. As argued by existentialist and humanist psychologists (e.g., Becker, 1973; May, 1958; Yalom, 1980), our lives are characterized by a basic conflict between "the awareness of the inevitability of death and the wish to continue to be" (Yalom, 1980, p. 8). As a result, the task of a fully functioning individual is not to suppress death anxiety but, rather, to accept and tolerate it, and forge an authentic existence that incorporates death awareness into the fabric of being. The dread of death is so powerful, however, argue the existentialists, that only a select few (the self-actualized) are capable of confronting it, with the majority of people relying on ritual, social roles and values to provide order and meaning in life and "anesthetize" against the terror of death anxiety (Becker, 1973; McCoy, Pyszczynski, Solomon, & Greenberg, 2000). Empirical support for the "morbid view" comes primarily from clinical case studies (Firestone, 1994; Maslow, 1967, 1976; Yalom, 1980).

Until now, no attempt has been made to reconcile the "healthy" and the "morbid" views of death anxiety which are treated as mutually exclusive (Firestone, 1994; Tomer & Eliason, 2000). This study attempts to bridge this dichotomy by drawing on Maslow's (1970) distinction between self-actualized individuals who are "peakers" (i.e., experience feelings of awe, transcendence, and merger with a larger force) and "non-peakers." Whereas peakers emphasize creativity, personal growth, and non-institutionalized forms of religious experiences, "non-peakers" value the practicality of everyday life, worldly success, and tradition (Maslow, 1970). Other scholars have proposed a similar dichotomy between personality types or modes of functioning such as the distinction between the introvert and extravert (Jung, 1921, 1976), the adapted and creative (artistic) individual (Rank, 1932), and object (other) and self-directedness (Blatt & Shichman, 1983; Wink, 1991). According to Rank (1932), for example, the adapted individual complies with tradition, experiences few conflicts, and emphasizes close relations with others. In contrast, the creative (artistic) individual places a premium on autonomy, seeks novel solutions to problems, and attempts to reconcile the fear of life associated with being separate from others (standing alone) and the fear of death related to union and dependence on others (see MacKinnon, 1965).

Implicit in Maslow's and Rank's dichotomies is the hypothesis that the self-actualized non-peaker or the adapted individual should experience low death anxiety because the conventionality associated with this personality type is expected to buffer against the fear of death and other negative emotions. Conversely, the self-actualized peaker or "artistic" individual who emphasizes personal growth and non-conventionality should be less strongly buffered against death anxiety. Further, if Maslow was correct in assuming that peakers and non-peakers exemplify different but equally adaptive forms of self-actualization, both should be characterized by positive psychosocial functioning in old age. In other words, the extension of Maslow's distinction to death studies suggests that there is more than one adaptive way of dealing with the fear of death depending on the individual's personality style. In this study, traditional and non-traditional forms of religiosity (religiousness and spirituality) were compared to test the hypothesis that there are two distinct ways of approaching death anxiety in old age.

RELIGIOUSNESS AND SPIRITUALITY

Since the cultural changes of the 1960s there has been a growing tendency in the United States to conceive of religiousness and spirituality as two distinct ways of relating to the sacred (e.g., Fuller, 2001; Marty, 1993). Whereas prior to the 1960s spiritual interests tended to be experienced within institutionalized religious traditions, since then a growing number of Americans engage in individualized spiritual practices that are generally outside the domain of religious institutions (Roof, 1999: Wuthnow, 1998). As a result, Wuthnow (1998) distinguishes between "religious dwellers" who tend to accept traditional religious practices and authority, and "spiritual seekers" for whom individual autonomy takes precedence over external authority and the hold of tradition-centered religious doctrines and practices. Unlike religious dwellers, spiritual seekers place a greater emphasis on self-growth, and typically emphasize the importance of experiencing a sense of integrated connection in everyday life with God, a higher power, and/or nature (Underwood, 1999: 12).

Spirituality can be defined in many diverse ways (Moberg, 2002), and, as argued by Pargament (1999), many researchers and lay persons tend to identify it as a central component of any religious experience. Following Wuthnow (1998), we have operationalized religiousness in terms of a religious orientation associated with institutionalized or tradition-centered religious practices and spirituality as a more privatized quest associated with involvement in non-institutionalized religious practices (Wink & Dillon, 2003). We decided to conceptualize religiousness and spirituality as two relatively independent dimensions because of our interest in contrasting the psychosocial implications of newer and more traditional forms of religious practices.

There are two reasons why the differentiation between religiousness and spirituality is particularly apt for testing the hypothesis that there are alternative ways of successfully coping with death anxiety. First, in past research, we have found that both religiousness and spirituality were related to positive aging (e.g., a generative concern for the welfare of others [Dillon, Wink, & Fay, 2003]). Second, similar to Maslow's self-actualized non-peaker and Rank's adapted type, individuals high in religiousness tend to value close relations with others, communal involvement (Wink & Dillon, 2003) and conventionality (Wink & Ciciolla, 2005) and, therefore, they should be buffered against the experience of negative emotions in general and of fear of death in particular. In contrast, spiritual seekers, just like self-actualized peakers and the artistic type, tend to emphasize personal growth (Wink & Dillon, 2003) and openness to experience (Wink & Ciciolla, 2005), and as a result should be more receptive in acknowledging death anxiety.

Hypotheses

Following Maslow (1970), it was hypothesized that in late adulthood both religiousness and spirituality should be associated with self-actualization operationalized as an achieved or integrated sense of personal identity and vital engagement in everyday life (Hypothesis 1). Only religiousness was expected, however, to be associated with an accepting identity (Helson, Stewart, & Ostrove, 1995)–characterized by conservative values and an internally consistent personality–and the presence of positive affect (life satisfaction). In contrast, only spirituality was anticipated to be related to a searching identity characterized by non-conformance and a concern with life's meaning, creativity, and, a tendency to reminisce which expresses an interest in personal growth (Hypothesis 2).

The third hypothesis concerned the relation among religiousness, spirituality, and the fear of death. Several studies report a linear negative relation between religion and the fear of death, meaning that high scores on religiousness are associated with low scores on fear of death and, conversely, low scores on religiousness are associated with an elevated fear of death (*the linear hypothesis*; Fortner & Neimeyer, 1999). Other studies indicate, however, that a low fear of death is a function of consistency between religious beliefs and practices (*the consistency hypothesis*; e.g., Leming, 1979-1980; Nelson & Cantrell, 1980) rather than being simply a linear correlate of strength of religious beliefs or intensity of religious practices. Based on previous findings from this sample (Wink & Scott, 2005), it was hypothesized that a low fear of death would characterize participants who showed consistency between their religious practices and their self-reported belief in a rewarding afterlife.

In contrast to religiousness, there is virtually no research on the relation between spirituality and fear of death with the exception of a study that found no relation between paranormal beliefs (e.g., belief in reincarnation, astral projection, witchcraft, and clairvoyance) and death anxiety (Tobacyk, 1984). In this study, it was hypothesized that spirituality would not be related (either linearly or as a function of consistency between spiritual practices and belief in an afterlife) to the fear of death. Although the openness to experience and interest in personal growth associated with spirituality should be conducive to the experience of death anxiety, a high level of self-realization should dampen an undue concern with mortality.

METHOD

Participants

The data came from the Intergenerational Studies established by the Institute of Human Development (IHD) at the University of California, Berkeley in the 1920s. The original sample was a representative sample of infants born in Berkeley (California) in 1928/29 (the Berkeley Guidance Study), and of pre-adolescents (ages 10-12) selected from elementary schools in Oakland (California) in 1931 and who were born in 1920/21 (the Oakland Growth Study). Both samples were combined into a single study in the 1960s (Eichorn, 1981). The participants were studied intensively in childhood and adolescence and interviewed in-depth four times in adulthood. In the present study, I used only data collected between 1997 and 2000 when the participants were in late adulthood (age late 60s or mid-70s). Prior analyses indicated very little bias due to sample attrition other than a slight tendency for lower participation rates among individuals with lower levels of education (Clausen, 1993; Wink & Dillon, 2002).

In this study, the *N* consisted of 155 participants who, in addition to being personally interviewed (*N* = 181), completed a self-report questionnaire that included measures of fear of death and of belief in the afterlife. A comparison of the participants who were interviewed and completed the questionnaire (*N* = 155) with those who were personally interviewed but who did not complete a questionnaire (*N* = 26) revealed no differences in religiousness, spirituality, social class, gender, or cohort.

In the current sample, 53% are women and 47% are men; 36% were born in the early 1920s and 64% were born in the late 1920s. All but 6 of the participants are White, reflecting the small fraction of non-Caucasians in the Bay Area in the 1920s when the sample was drawn. Forty-seven percent were college graduates. In late middle adulthood, 59% of the participants (or their spouses) were upper middle class professionals or executives, 19% were lower middle class, and 22% were working class. In late adulthood, 71% (85% of men and 55% of women) were living with their spouse or partner. The majority of the sample (73%) grew up in Protestant families; 16% grew up Catholic, 5% grew up in mixed religious households, and 6% came from non-religious families. In late adulthood, 45% reported weekly church attendance and 81% said that religion was important in their lives. These figures closely parallel national polls; 52% of Americans in the 65 to 74 age category attend church weekly and 90% say that religion is important in their lives (Gallup & Lindsay, 1999).

Measures

Death Attitudes were assessed with the self-report Death Attitudes Profile (DAP; Gesser, Wong, & Reker, 1987-1988) administered to the IHD participants in late adulthood. The *Fear of Death* scale measures anxiety associated with the prospect of death (e.g., "The prospect of my own death arouses anxiety in me.") (see Wink & Scott, 2005). The *Belief in Afterlife* scale reflects the view of death as a passageway to a happy afterlife (e.g., "I see death as a passage to an eternal and blessed place.") (Gesser et al., 1987-1988). The alpha reliability for the Fear of Death scale was .82, and for the Belief in Afterlife scale was .91.

Religiousness and spirituality were coded on separate 5-point scales independently by two raters using responses to structured open-ended questions on religious beliefs and practices from transcripts of interviews conducted with the participants in late adulthood.

Religiousness was operationalized as the importance of traditional or institutionalized religious beliefs and practices in the life of the individual. A score of 5 indicated that religious beliefs (e.g., belief in God) and practices (e.g., church attendance and prayer) played a *central* role in the respondent's life. A score of 3 indicated that religious beliefs and practices had *some* importance in the individual's life, and a score of 1 indicated that religion played *no part* in the life of the individual. Our measure of belief in a rewarding afterlife did not assume engagement in religious practices, and, conversely, the study's measure of religiousness was skewed toward the importance of everyday practice. Thus although religiousness and belief in an afterlife were highly intercorrelated (see the Results section), they are conceptually distinct.

Spirituality was operationalized as the importance of nontraditional or deinstitutionalized religious beliefs and practices in the life of the individual. A score of 5 indicated that non-institutionalized religion or non-tradition-centered religious beliefs and practices played a *central* role in the individual's life. The person typically reported a sense of sacred connectedness with God, a Higher Power, or nature, and systematically engaged in spiritual practices (e.g., meditation, Shamanistic journeying, centering, or contemplative prayer) on a regular basis. A score of 3 indicated that spirituality had *some* importance in the life of the individual; the individual reported spiritual experiences and engaged in occasional spiritual practices. A score of 1 indicated that the individual reported *no interest* in spiritual matters.

In late adulthood, the Kappa index of reliability was .72 for the ratings of religiousness, and .63 for the rating of spirituality. Religiousness and spirituality were moderately intercorrelated ($r(155) = .36, p < .01$).

Identity. The identity statuses of the IHD participants were assessed using the California Adult Q-set (CAQ; Block, 1971). This observer-based, ipsative procedure enables trained expert raters to describe the personality and social behavior of the interviewee using a deck of 100 sentence descriptors that raters sort into nine forced-choice categories ranging from extremely characteristic to extremely uncharacteristic. Independent panels of between two and four raters used the interview material from the late adulthood interviews to provide composite CAQ ratings for each participant. The CAQ *Integrated (Achieved) Identity* scale consisted of 12 CAQ items judged by a panel of experts to be most characteristic of the construct (Mallory, 1989). It assesses a mature sense of self or an integrated identity that reflects a balance between agency, interpersonal relations, and personal values (Marcia, 1966; Helson et al., 1995). CAQ items representative of the Integrated Identity scale are: "Is productive; get things done," "Has warmth, capacity for close relationships," "Behaves in an ethically consistent manner."

The *CAQ Searching (Moratorium) Identity* scale consisted of 9 CAQ items judged by experts to reflect a sense of identity based on a questioning stance towards the social environment (e.g., "Is introspective," "Tends to be rebellious and non-conforming," and "Is concerned with philosophical problems and meaning in life." The *CAQ Accepting (Foreclosed) Identity* scale consisted of 10 CAQ items judged by experts to reflect a sense of identity based on an acceptance of social norms and values (e.g., "Favors conservative values in a variety of areas," "Is moralistic," "Has a clear-cut, internally consistent personality") (Mallory, 1969; Helson et al., 1995). Cronbach's alpha coefficients of reliability for the Integrated, Searching, and Accepting Identity scales were .81, .62, and .72, respectively.

Personality functioning was assessed with two scales from the California Psychological Inventory (CPI; Gough & Bradley, 2003), a widely used self-report personality test. The *Norm-Favoring* scale is a measure of a conventional, conservative, and norm-abiding mode of adaptation (Gough & Bradley, 2003). The *Creative Temperament* scale is a measure of a personality style characterized by adventurousness, unconventionality, and spontaneity (Gough, 1992).

Level of involvement in everyday life tasks was the sum total of scores on the six scales of Harlow and Cantor's (1996) self-report *Life Task Participation scale* (alpha = .79). The scale measured daily involvement in six domains: social activities, reading and watching mass media, increasing knowledge or building skills, home activities or hobbies, creative activities, activities outside home (e.g., travel and participating in sports), and community service activities. *Positive Reminiscence* was assessed as the sum total of scores on six out of eight scales of the self-report Reminiscence Functions scale (RFS; Webster, 1993) (alpha = .95). Items in the scale included the use of reminiscence for the purpose of death preparation, identity exploration, problem-solving, conversation, intimacy maintenance, and teaching or informing. (Excluded from the measure were two RFS subscales assessing a negative use of reminiscence for the purpose of bitterness revival and boredom reduction.) *Life satisfaction* was measured with the 5-point Satisfaction with Life Scale (Diener, Emmons, Larsen, & Griffin, 1985) (Cronbach's *alpha* = .90).

RESULTS

Religiousness, Spirituality, and Psychosocial Functioning in Late Adulthood

Religiousness and spirituality were correlated with an array of characteristics in late adulthood in order to test their relation with psychosocial functioning. In view of the moderately positive relation between religiousness and spirituality, these analyses were replicated using partial correlations in order to establish the relation between religiousness and psychosocial functioning when its overlap with spirituality was removed, and, conversely, to ascertain the relation between spirituality and psychosocial functioning when its overlap with religiousness was removed.

As hypothesized, both religiousness and spirituality were positively related to self-actualization indicated by participation in everyday life tasks and an integrated sense of identity (see Table 1). Only religiousness was positively related to an accepting identity, identification with social norms, and life satisfaction. In contrast, only spirituality was positively related to a searching identity, creative temperament, and the positive use of reminiscence. (In the case of religiousness, its correlation with positive reminiscence became insignificant after spirituality was partialled out.)

Relation Between Religiousness and Spirituality and Death Attitudes

Both religiousness and spirituality were positively related to the belief in a rewarding afterlife (r (155) = .70 and .36, $p < .01$, respectively). Neither correlated, however, with fear of death (r (155) = $-.06$ for religiousness, and r (155) = $-.10$ for spirituality). Separate two-way ANOVAs were performed to test the hypothesis that fear of death (the dependent variable) would be lowest among participants who showed congruence between belief in an afterlife and religiousness or, alternatively, spirituality. Religiousness, Spirituality, and Belief in Afterlife were converted to dummy 1/0 variables so that they could be used as independent variables in the ANOVAs.[1] Spirituality was used as a covariate in the ANOVA in which religiousness was the predictor of fear of death and, conversely, religiousness was used as a covariate in the ANOVA in which spirituality was the predictor.

TABLE 1. Relation Between Religiousness, Spirituality, and Psychological Functioning in Late Adulthood

Characteristics in Late Adulthood	Religiousness		Spirituality	
	r	Partial r	s	Partial s
Common to Religiousness and Spirituality				
Life Task Participation	.28**	.22*	.24**	.29**
Integrated Identity	.30**	.21*	.27**	.18**
More Typical of Religiousness				
Accepting Identity	.22*	.34**	−.30**	.39**
Norm Favoring Personality	.26**	.30**	−.07	−.17
Life Satisfaction	.17*	.18*	.02	−.04
More Typical of Spirituality				
Searching Identity	.00	−.18*	.49**	.51**
Creative Temperament	−.08	−.19*	.30**	.24**
Positive Reminiscence	.24*	.15	.28**	.22*

N = 155 for all measures with the exception of Norm Favoring Personality and Creative Temperament (N = 121), and Positive Reminiscence (N = 117).
*p < .05; **p < .01.

In the two-way ANOVA predicting fear of death from religiousness and belief in an afterlife, the two main effects were not significant ($F(1,152)$ = .18 and .00 for religiousness and belief in an afterlife, respectively). There was, however, a significant two-way interaction between religiousness and belief in an afterlife ($F(1,152)$ = 5.75, p < .01). As shown in Figure 1, the interaction was significant because, as hypothesized, participants who were high in both religiousness and belief in afterlife were less afraid of death than the two inconsistent groups (high religiousness and low belief in afterlife and low religiousness and high belief in afterlife). In addition, a low fear of death was also characteristic of individuals who were low in both religiousness and belief in afterlife (see also Wink & Scott, 2005).

Follow-up analyses indicated that among individuals who reported a high belief in afterlife, those who were high in religiousness (the consistent religious group) scored significantly lower on fear of death than those who were low in religiousness ($t(28,50)$ = 2.16, p < .05). Conversely, among participants who reported a low belief in afterlife, those

FIGURE 1. The Religiousness × Belief in Afterlife interaction is significant.

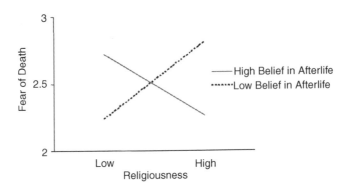

who were low in religiousness (the consistent non-religious group) tended to be less afraid of death than those who were high in religiousness ($t(69,8) = -1.75; p = .08$).

In the second two-way ANOVA predicting fear of death from spirituality and belief in an afterlife, the main effects ($F(1.152) = 1.82$, and $F(1,152) = .02$) of belief in afterlife and spirituality, respectively) were not significant. Neither was the two-way interaction ($F(1,152) = .63$) significant (see Figure 2). In other words, spirituality on its own or in combination with a belief in afterlife did not act as a buffer against fear of death.

DISCUSSION

This study investigated the relation among religiousness, spirituality, and fear of death in order to test the hypothesis that there are two distinct ways of successfully managing death anxiety in old age. As expected, religiousness in late adulthood served as a buffer against fear of death. This relation proved to be more complicated, however, than assumed by the linear hypothesis because there was no significant correlation between religiousness and fear of death. In other words, high scores on religiousness (when considered on their own) were not associated with low fear of death and, conversely, low scores on religiousness did not imply an elevated fear of death. Instead, religiousness and belief in a re-

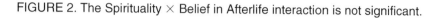

FIGURE 2. The Spirituality × Belief in Afterlife interaction is not significant.

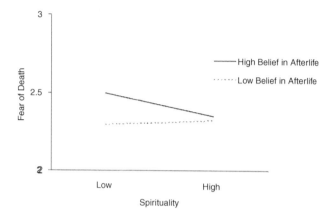

warding afterlife interacted in predicting death anxiety. The study participants who showed a consistency between high levels of religious beliefs and practices were less afraid of death than participants who lacked such consistency. The same was also true of individuals who scored consistently low on religiousness and belief in afterlife. In other words, it is the *consistency* between one's views on death and related behavior that buffers against death anxiety in late adulthood. Conversely, lack of such consistency appears to predispose the individual to fear of death. This finding replicates that of Wink and Scott (2005), obtained using the same data set but a different statistical procedure (i.e., linear multiple regression analysis as opposed to ANOVA).

In contrast to religiousness, spirituality was not related to fear of death either in the analysis testing for a linear relation or in the analysis testing for an interaction between spirituality and belief in a rewarding afterlife (the consistency hypothesis). In other words, spirituality and fear of death were not related in any consistent manner that was discernible in this study. Why was this the case? It could be argued that if consistency buffers against the fear of death, then belief in an afterlife may be an inappropriate measure to test for congruence between the beliefs and practices of highly spiritual individuals. Although spirituality was positively related to belief in an afterlife, the magnitude of this relation was considerably lower than for religiousness. Belief in an afterlife is clearly not as central to spiritual seeking as it is to religiousness despite the fact that many spiritual individuals believe in reincarnation and other forms of continued existence after death. It is unclear, however, what other characteristics could be used to test the consistency hypothesis for spirituality.

Another explanation why spirituality was not related to fear of death focuses attention on the notion of consistency itself. It could be argued that consistency between beliefs and practices, irrespective of whether it is based on a secular or sacred ideology, buffers against fear of death because it signals a conventionality or congruence of personality that is characteristic of Rank's (1932) adapted individual, of Maslow's (1970) self-actualized non-peaker, and of the "healthy view" of death anxiety. If this is the case, then spiritual individuals whose identity is characterized by non-conventionality and a quest for meaning may not place a premium on personal consistency. Alternatively, consistency may have different implications for the functioning of spiritual individuals than for persons who are high in religiousness.

Irrespective of the reason, the absence of a positive relation between spirituality and fear of death raises the question whether highly spiritual older adults exemplify the same level of self-realization as their counterparts who are high in religiousness. Or, alternatively, is spiritual seeking, as suggested by cultural critics (e.g., Bellah, Madsen, Sullivan, Swidler, & Tipton, 1985; Lasch, 1979; Rieff, 1966) reflective of a fragile self and an ad hoc therapeutic desire to fix emotional problems without the disciplined commitment typically associated with more traditional forms of religiousness? The positive relation between both spirituality and religiousness and self-actualization–an integrated identity and vital involvement in everyday activities–does not support this second interpretation. In other words, highly spiritual individuals, similar to individuals high in religiousness, appear to possess adequate personal resources and discipline for positive psychosocial functioning.

The results from this study suggest that religiousness and spirituality reflect two different pathways to successful aging–one characterized by a more conventional and the other by a more unconventional mode of functioning. For individuals who are consistent in their religious beliefs and practices, the absence of fear of death fits well with their high level of life satisfaction and identification with a norm-abiding mode of adaptation. In the case of spirituality, a lack of relation with fear of death reflects an emphasis on openness to experience associated with creativity and personal growth. These two modes of psychosocial functioning appear to be adaptive to the demands of older adulthood and, in particular, to the older age individual's negotiation of death anxiety.

For the clinical practitioner, these findings suggest that the meaning of the presence or absence of fear of death in older age clients can be only established against the backdrop of their overall mode of psychosocial functioning. A highly spiritual individual may, for example, respond to personal adversity or the aging process more generally by acknowledging death anxiety in an appropriate way as part of a personal journey of self-discovery. In contrast, for an individual who is high in religiousness even a moderate amount of fear of death may be a sign of difficulties in coping or adjustment. Clinicians should be sensitive to both these possibilities and apply appropriate standards in assessing the significance of death anxiety, standards that respect different ways in which an individual composes his or her life and deals with its vicissitudes.

Finally, it is important to acknowledge the limitations of the present study. The sample consisted of white Christians who were born in Northern California in the 1920s. In addition, the precise nature of the differentiation between religiousness and spirituality is both a subject of theoretical debate and is hard to assess quantitatively. The findings of this study need to be replicated in samples with a greater diversity of age, race, and religious affiliation and using other measures of religiousness and spirituality. Nonetheless, it is hoped that the present results will add both to the understanding of the nature of death anxiety and stimulate discussion of its management in the lives of the elderly.

NOTE

1. For religiousness 1 = a score of 3 or above on the 5-point rating of religiousness; for spirituality a score of 1 = 2.5 or above on the 5-point rating of spirituality, and for belief in afterlife 1 = a mean score or above on the DAP Belief in a Rewarding Afterlife scale. A slightly lower cut-off point was used for spirituality compared to religiousness because fewer participants scored high on spirituality.

REFERENCES

Becker, E. (1973). *The denial of death*. New York: Free Press.

Bellah, R., Madsen, R., Sullivan, W., Swidler, A., & Tipton, S. (1985). *Habits of the heart: Individualism and commitment in American life*. Berkeley, CA: University of California Press.

Blatt, S., & Shichman, S. (1983). Two primary configurations of psychopathology. *Psychoanalysis and Contemporary Thought, 6*, 187-254.

Block, J. (1971). *Lives through time* (2nd ed.). Berkeley, CA: Bancroft.

Clausen, J. (1993). *American lives*. New York: Free Press.

Diener, E., Emmons, R. A., Larsen, R. J., & Griffin, S. (1985). The satisfaction with life scale. *Journal of Personality Assessment, 49*, 71-75.

Dillon, M., Wink, P., & Fay, K. (2003). Is spirituality detrimental to generativity? *Journal for the Scientific Study of Religion, 42*, 427-442.

Eichorn, D. (1981). Samples and procedure. In D. Eichorn, J. A. Clausen, N. Haan, M. P. Honzik, & P. H. Mussen (Eds.), *Present and past in middle life* (pp. 33-51). New York: Academic Press.

Erikson, E. H. (1963). *Childhood and society*. New York: Norton.

Firestone, R. W. (1994). Psychological defenses against death anxiety. In R. A. Neimeyer (Ed.), *Death anxiety handbook: Research, instrumentation, and application* (pp. 217-241). Washington, DC: Taylor & Francis.

Fortner, B. V., & Neimeyer, R. A. (1999). Death anxiety in older adults: A quantitative review. *Death Studies, 23*, 387-411.

Fuller, R. C. (2001). *Spiritual, but not religious*. New York: Oxford University Press.

Gallup, G., & Lindsay, D. M. (1999). *Surveying the religious landscape*. Harrisburg, PA: Morehouse.

Gesser, G., Wong, P. T. P., & Reker, G. T. (1987-88). Death attitudes across the life-span: The development and validation of the Death Attitude Profile (DAP). *Omega, 18*, 109-124.

Goodman, (1981). *Death and the creative life*. New York: Springer.

Gough, H. G. (1992). Assessment of creative potential in psychology and the development of a creative temperament scale for the CPI. In J. C. Rosen & P. McReynolds (Eds.), *Advances in psychological assessment, 8*, 227-259. New York: Plenum.

Gough, H. G., & Bradley, P. (2003). *California psychological inventory manual* (4th ed.). Palo Alto, CA: Consulting Psychologists Press.

Harlow, R., & Cantor, N. (1996). Still participating after all these years: A study of life task participation in later life. *Journal of Personality & Social Psychology, 71*, 1235-1249.

Helson, R., Stewart, A. J., Ostrove, J. (1995). Identity in three cohorts of midlife women. *Journal of Personality & Social Psychology, 69*, 544-557.

Jung, C. G. (1976). *Psychological types*. Princeton, NJ: Princeton University Press. (Original work published 1921.)

Kubler-Ross, (1997). *The wheel of life: A memoir of living and dying*. New York: Simon & Schuster.

Lasch, C. 1979. *The culture of narcissism: American life in an age of diminishing expectations*. New York: Norton.

Leming, M. R. (1979-80). Religion and death: A test of Homans' thesis. *Omega, 10*, 1979-80.

Loretto, R., & Templer, D. I. (1986). *Death anxiety*. New York: Hemisphere.

MacKinnon, D. W. (1965). Personality and the realization of creative potential. *American Psychologist, 20*, 273-281.

Mallory, M. E. (1989). Q-sort definition of ego identity status. *Journal of Youth & Adolescence, 18*, 399-412.

Marcia, J. E. (1966). Development and validation of ego identity status. *Journal of Personality & Social Psychology, 3*, 551-558.

Marty, M. (1993). Where the energies go. *Annals of the American Academy of Political and Social Science, 553,* 11-26.

Maslow, A. H. (1970). *Motivation and personality* (2nd ed.). New York: Harper & Row.

Maslow, A. H. (1976). *The farther reaches of human nature.* New York: Penguin. (Original work published 1967).

May, R. (1958). Contributions of existential psychotherapy. In R. May, E. Angel, & H. F. Ellenberger (Eds.), *Existence; A new dimension in psychiatry and psychology* (37-91). New York: Simon and Schuster.

McCoy, S. K., Pyszczynski, T., Solomon, S., & Greenberg, J. (2000). Transcending the self: A terror management perspective on successful aging. In A. Tomer (Ed.), *Death attitudes and the older adult* (pp. 37-64). Washington, DC: Taylor & Francis.

Moberg, D. (2002). Assessing and measuring spirituality: Confronting dilemmas of universal and particular evaluative criteria. *Journal of Adult Development, 9,* 47-60.

Neimeyer, R. A., & Van Brunt, D. (1995). Death anxiety. In H. Wass, & R. A. Neimeyer (Eds.), *Dying: Facing the facts* (3rd ed., 49-87). Boston, MA: Taylor & Francis.

Nelson, L. D., & Cantrell, C. H. (1980). Religiosity and death anxiety: A multi-dimensional analysis. *Review of Religious Research, 21,* 148-157.

Pargament, K. I. (1999). The psychology of religion and spirituality? Yes and no. *International Journal for the Psychology of Religion, 9,* 3-16.

Rank, O. (1932). *Art and artist: Creative urge and personality development.* New York: Knopf.

Rieff, P. (1966). *The triumph of the therapeutic: Uses of faith after Freud.* New York: Harper & Row.

Roof, W. C. (1999). *Spiritual marketplace: Baby boomers and the remaking of American religion.* Princeton, NJ: Princeton University Press.

Tobacyk, J. (1984). Death threat, death concerns, and paranormal belief. In F. R. Epting & R. A. Neimeyer (Eds.), *Personal meanings of death: Applications of personal construct theory to clinical practice* (29-41). Washington, DC: Hemisphere Publishing.

Tomer, A., & Eliason, G. (2000). Attitudes about life and death. In A. Tomer (Ed.), *Death attitudes and the older adult* (3-22). Washington, DC: Taylor & Francis.

Underwood, L. (1999). Daily spiritual experiences. In *Multidimensional measurement of religiousness/spirituality for use in health research* (11-17). Kalamazoo, MI: John E. Fetzer Institute.

Webster, J. D. (1993). Construction and validation of the reminiscence functions scale. *Journal of Gerontology: Psychological Sciences, 48,* 256-262.

Wink, P. (1991). Self and object-directedness in middle-aged women. *Journal of Personality, 59,* 769-791.

Wink, P., & Ciciolla, L. (2005). *Relation between religiousness, spirituality, and personality: Findings from a long-term longitudinal study.* Unpublished manuscript, Wellesley College, Wellesley.

Wink, P., & Dillon, M. 2002. Spiritual development across the adult life course: Findings from a longitudinal study. *Journal of Adult Development, 9,* 79-94.

Wink, P., & Dillon, M. (2003). Religiousness, spirituality, and psychosocial functioning in late adulthood: Findings from a longitudinal study. *Psychology and Aging, 18,*
916-924.

Wink, P., & Scott, J. (2005). Does religiousness buffer against the fear of death and dying in late adulthood? Findings from a longitudinal study. *Journal of Gerontology:
Psychological Sciences, 60B,* 207-214.

Wong, P. T. P., Reker, G. T., & Gesser, T. (1994). *Death attitude profile–Revised: A
multidimensional measure of attitudes toward death.* In R. A. Neimeyer (Ed.),
Death anxiety handbook (121-148). Washington, DC: Taylor & Francis.

Wong, P. T. P. (2000). Meaning of life and meaning of death in successful aging. In A.
Tomer (Ed.), *Death attitudes and the older adult* (pp. 23-35). Washington, DC: Taylor &
Francis.

Wuthnow, R. 1998. *After heaven: Spirituality in America since the 1950s.* Berkeley: University of California Press.

Yalom, I. (1980). *Existential psychotherapy.* New York: Basic Books.

The Pain of Dying

Michael Barbato, MBBS, FRACP

SUMMARY. Dying can be a painful and difficult business. Fears, hopes, losses, questions, and uncertainty result in a form of pain that lies beyond the therapeutic reach of science and pharmacology. Efforts to preserve and prolong life or to make things better can sometimes result in this pain being overlooked or remaining unheard. To search the deepest part of oneself is the journey that beckons us all as we are dying. Within this space resides the source of our own suffering but also the seeds for healing. This exploration has a momentum of its own but requires conditions not often found within the biomedical paradigm. If this model of care remains the only source of hope for those with a life-threatening illness, 'the pain of dying' may not be addressed. *[Article copies available for a fee from The Haworth Document Delivery Service: 1-800-HAWORTH. E-mail address: <docdelivery@haworthpress.com> Website: <http://www.HaworthPress.com> ©2006 by The Haworth Press, Inc. All rights reserved.]*

KEYWORDS. Dying, suffering, pain, metaphor, healing, healthcare

---

Michael Barbato, MBBS, FRACP, is affiliated with the Conscious Living Conscious Dying Centre, 91 Barney Street, Kiama NSW 2533, Australia (E-mail: barbato@iimetro.com.au).

[Haworth co-indexing entry note]: "The Pain of Dying." Barbato, Michael. Co-published simultaneously in *Journal of Religion, Spirituality & Aging* (The Haworth Pastoral Press, an imprint of The Haworth Press, Inc.) Vol. 18, No. 2/3, 2006, pp. 111-122; and: *Aging, Spirituality and Palliative Care* (ed: Elizabeth MacKinlay) The Haworth Pastoral Press, an imprint of The Haworth Press, Inc., 2006, pp. 111-122. Single or multiple copies of this article are available for a fee from The Haworth Document Delivery Service [1-800-HAWORTH, 9:00 a.m. - 5:00 p.m. (EST). E-mail address: docdelivery@haworthpress.com].

The intuitive mind is a sacred gift and the rational mind a faithful servant. We have created a society that honours the servant and has forgotten the gift.

Albert Einstein

INTRODUCTION

Despite 40 years of clinical practice (including the last 15 years in palliative medicine), I feel ill-equipped to unravel the mysteries and vicissitudes that surround death and dying. In saying this I am reminded of and take heart from the story of the Zen master who when asked by a student to tell him about death said that he knew nothing about the topic. "How can that be so," said the student, "a master must surely have knowledge of such things?" To which the master replied, "ah, but I am not a dead Zen master."

As a palliative care physician I have cared for many people in their final days, weeks, or months of life but that experience has not brought me any closer to really appreciating what it may be like to die. Indeed I believe there is a real danger in palliative care that experience, measured in years, can lead to a distancing rather than an understanding of a patient's suffering. A North American Indian proverb states "in order to truly understand a man, one must walk a mile in his moccasins." This saying reminds us of the quantum difference that exists between the objective and subjective experience and the danger in extrapolating from observation alone. But, given the fact I am alive and healthy I have no recourse but to offer observations based on my life's experience and clinical practice supplemented at times with stories and quotations from those who have died.

Those familiar with the palliative care literature would know there is no shortage of terms to describe the pain of dying. Words such as suffering, spiritual pain, existential pain and soul pain are but a few (Cassell, 1982; Kearney, 1996; Saunders, 1988; Strang et al., 2004). The struggle to find a suitable term not only indicates the difficulty in defining such pain, it also reminds us how 'painfully' inadequate words are when used to describe an experience such as dying. For this reason, metaphors, similes, and analogies are frequently used to express what ordinary language alone cannot. These vehicles for expression are a "linguistic anchor for our confused attempts to understand a potentially ineffable phenomenon" (Barker, 2000). They help our mind process the unprocessable, comprehend the incomprehensible and speak the unspeakable.

Philippe Ariès in his landmark text *The Hour of Our Death* (Ariès, 1981, p. 410) says "adults are afraid of death as children are afraid of the dark." These are more than mere words. The analogy takes us beyond the rational analytical mind which cannot conceive something as abstract as death and uses a life event that is familiar, knowable and emotive to communicate the essence of the death experience, i.e., the fear of the unknown. Bridging the heart-mind gap allows us to identify at some deeper feeling level with an otherwise unknowable experience.

Grahame Jones in his book *Magnanimous Despair* uses metaphor to vividly and graphically illustrate what it was like for him as he approached death. He says:

> I recall the little Dutch boy at the dyke cleverly holding back the mighty flood with his finger. I too feel like the little Dutch boy. With my hands I am reaching out to cover the cracks in the wall. But as I hold out at full stretch I do so with fear, the knowledge that another break will come somewhere beyond my reach and at a moment when both hands are engaged elsewhere. (Jones, 1998, p. 9)

Grahame's fear and uncertainty are brought to life with this metaphor. We can visualise his struggle, hear his pain, and sense his fear. As onlookers we are therefore better placed to empathise with him.

Visual imagery also adds a level of understanding not usually found in language alone. The adage, a picture is worth a thousand words, is particularly true when it comes to describing an emotional experience such as dying. A picture or television footage depicting tragedy in the life of an individual or community has a greater emotional impact than the words that accompany the story. We often forget what was said but the imagery lives on in our memory and emotions. The devastation and grief arising from the destruction of the World Trade Center in September 2001 (and the recent tsunami tragedy) illustrate this point.

The following examples do not have death as their subject but if used to symbolise death they become the visual equivalent of a metaphor and help us to better appreciate some aspects of dying that are otherwise incomprehensible. What we see and feel slips beneath the impenetrable skin of our understanding and resonates at some deeper and more profound level. The first is the painting 'Fisherman at Sea' by Joseph Turner and the other a photograph from the Sydney Catholic Education Office (CEO) photo-library depicting criss-crossing railway tracks. The foreground to the Joseph Turner painting is heavy and fearsome but the background of calmer waters and light is an implicit message of hope even at the darkest times. The symbolism with dying is very clear. The CEO photograph (Cooney & Burton, 1986) is a symbolic representation of the unpredictable and uncertain journey of the dying person and the numerous perplexing choices that have to be made.

No matter how extensive our experience or how good the description or the imagery, the pain of dying will however always be something we know of and not about. As healthy observers such pain is outside our immediate world. We can imagine but we cannot feel what it might be like to die. The difference between knowing and feeling is immeasurable and nothing other than direct experience can bridge that gap. Most of us have experienced love and know all too well how different that is to a simple knowledge of the subject. T.S. Eliot (1965, pp. 65-66) expresses it so, "however certain our expectations, the moment foreseen may be unexpected when it arrives." Or in the words of many of my patients, "I never thought it would be like this."

THE PAIN OF DYING

Henry Thoreau was not the first person to challenge the widely held belief that happiness is the prerogative of us all. His poignant reflection (1966, p. 12), "people lead lives of quiet desperation," is a sad commentary on life, one that most of us would prefer to reject. It does, however, have a ring of truth when we consider the life of those who are dying. Certainly there are individuals who, by virtue of their age, beliefs or life practises are not afraid of death and approach it with an equanimity that most of us would find hard to believe. These people not only resign themselves to the inevitability of dying but accept it graciously and in some cases welcome it. For the majority, however, there is anguish, pain and suffering, much of which is indescribable, unfathomable, and often unreachable even though it dominates their life. Indeed much of their suffering results from the fact that what dying people feel is surreal and beyond belief. Their life takes on the guise of a nightmare from which they hope to awaken. This struggle to find the connection between what they feel on the inside with what is happening on the outside is the desperation that Thoreau talks of and what John of the Cross and St. Teresa of Avila call "a dark night of the soul."

How can a person talk about a pain that is heartfelt, multi-dimensional, and where there are no words to truly describe it? Mavis had been admitted to the local palliative care unit because of pain secondary to advanced malignancy. Pain control was achieved with little difficulty but depression and withdrawal evident at the time of admission had become more profound. Counselling and pharmacological interventions were marginally helpful but Mavis remained tormented and was unable to connect with or verbalise her deepest feelings. Reluctantly she agreed to attend an art therapy class where one of the tasks that day was to draw an apple. Much to the therapist's surprise, Mavis quietly engaged the activity, but rather than draw the apple, she drew an apple core. Later she revealed how this image put her in touch with overwhelming grief. She had for the first time found an image that helped her connect what was happening on the inside. She could now 'see' how the cancer was destroying her body as well as her life and this resonated strongly with the grief she felt. This unexpected realization was a turning point for her. She opened to the feelings in her heart, which until that time had all but paralysed her. What she had drawn was the metaphorical food that provided substance for reflection, exploration and dialogue. It was a healing experience.

According to Phil Barker it is very difficult to make any meaningful statement about oneself without recourse to metaphor (Barker, 1999).Those who cannot find words to describe their pain or how they feel not uncommonly resort to metaphor or simile. A young woman dying of cancer described her body as though "wrapped in barbed wire." Not infrequently we hear dying patients say their life is a nightmare or their world has fallen apart, or they feel as if they have been hit by a bus, or they are at the end of the road, or they hope there is some light at the end of the tunnel. All very descriptive metaphors telling us in no uncertain terms how they feel. Another of my patients who for cultural reasons had not been told she was dying used the following symbolic message to gently and beautifully inform her family that she was aware of her fate: "my boat has come, my bags are packed, I am going on a beautiful holiday but none of you can come with me."

Because metaphor and symbolism is the language of those who are the dying, carers should be attuned to it and utilize it often when communicating with them. This is exactly what a colleague did when asked by one of his patients if he was dying. The patient was an ex-boxer and his poor education often meant he did not understand much of the medical jargon. He did, however, understand exactly what the doctor said when he answered his question as follows: "the bell has sounded for the last round."

Whether the pain is primarily physical, emotional, spiritual or existential, there is frequently a dualistic quality to it. We experience pain
because consciously or sub-consciously we are aware of what we have
lost or are about to lose. In the words of Kahlil Gibran, "when you are
sorrowful, look again in your heart, and you will see that in truth you are
weeping for that which has been your delight" (Gibran, 1979, p. 36).
The following statements made by people during the final days of their
life illustrate the dualistic nature of their suffering and the tensions they
are forced to bear.

- This is all so surreal. I feel pain, I struggle for my breath and I see
  my body wasting but I do not feel as if I am dying.
- I feel full of life, have the desire to live, but I am tired of a body
  whose very existence has been undermined on all fronts.
- I don't want to die but I don't want to live this way.
- I am not afraid of death but I do not want to leave you.
- Confrontation with the worst often leads me to get the best out of
  existence (Jones, 1998, p. 84).
- Because I can no longer ignore death I pay more attention to life
  (Wilber, 1991).

In his book *Dark Nights of the Soul,* Thomas Moore talks about
liminality, a state where a person feels they are living between two
places, the known and the unknown, the familiar and the unfamiliar
(Moore, 2004). The term most certainly applies to the space of dying
and highlights the dualistic nature of a patient's suffering. Table 1 lists
some of the tensions, or in Moore's words, the in-between places people
find themselves in during the course of a life-threatening illness. They
may, for example:

- wonder if they are living or dying
- try to remain rational although overwhelmed by emotions
- wish to cease treatment but fear the consequences
- value independence but know they cannot manage on their own
- live in hope but dread the future
- feel like surrendering but are given messages to keep fighting

While such dualities have always been part of the territory, medical
and technological advances over the last century have added to the list
of choices (Cassell, 1999). Death, according to Daniel Callahan, "is
now harder to predict, more difficult to manage, the source of more and

TABLE 1. Some In-Between Places Associated with Dying

Dying	Living
Remaining rational	Feeling emotional
Hospital/hospice	Home
No treatment	Treatment
Dependence	Autonomy
Despair	Meaning
Fears	Hopes
Unknown	Known
Letting go	Reaching out
Fighting	Surrendering
Indignity	Dignity
Rejection	Acceptance
Sadness	Gratitude

more moral dilemmas and nasty choices, and spiritually more productive of anguish, ambivalence, and uncertainty" (Callahan, 1993, p. 33). Speak to any person with a life-threatening illness and they will tell you about the seemingly endless number of decisions that need to be made, the uncertainties associated with such choices and the resulting impact on them and the various members of their family. No one disputes the valuable contribution made by medicine over the last 100 years but what Daniel Callahan is rightly questioning is the appropriateness of the bio-medical paradigm when a person is dying and where suffering extends far beyond the identified patient.

In this era of confidentiality and privacy, family and friends are often the neglected or forgotten people in a model of care that is patient and disease focused. They suffer and their suffering interfaces with and contributes to that of the dying person. In most cases this admixture of pain bubbles away but the lid, figuratively speaking, remains firmly closed. Patient and family suffer in silence and concerns for themselves and others are rarely shared. The disastrous consequence of such an approach is plainly evident in the statement, made by one of my patients as she herself was dying of bowel cancer, "it's not the cancer that is killing me but the way it is tearing my family apart."

HOW COMMON IS THE PAIN OF DYING?

For most but certainly not all people, dying is a painful experience. When someone receives a life-threatening diagnosis their life is forever changed. They live with uncertainty, the fear of death and in the case of cancer, the fear of a painful death. Perhaps the most unanticipated and devastating change, however, is to the person's way of life. Life often becomes a procession of symptoms, tests, treatments, decisions, visits to and visits by health professionals. They grieve for what they have lost, namely good health, independence, a secure future and what Grahame Jones refers to as precious normality. He says, "what I detest is how effectively the procedure of the treatment robs me of my precious normality and seriously affects my morale" (Jones, 1998, p. 35). It is not surprising then to know that psychological and existential concerns are more prevalent than physical symptoms in those with a life-threatening illness (Portenoy et al., 1994).

In a survey of 248 cancer patients asked the question 'what are your most important needs,' Moadel found that help with overcoming fear was the most frequent described need followed by peace of mind and guidance to find hope, meaning, and spiritual resources (Moadel et al., 1999). Sadly, in real life, cancer patients are rarely asked the question 'what are your most important needs' nor do they have time to reflect on or discuss such important issues. While we in clinical practice espouse holistic care, the overriding emphasis is on the physical dimension often at the expense of all else (Cassell, 1999). From one who has personal experience, Grahame Jones reflects, "it does seem bitterly sad that my fate, the fate of me, will be decided, indirectly, through the functioning of a fleshly envelope. I see the soul, thus entrapped, as being the great and ultimate casualty of cancer's mortal war" (Jones, 1998, p. 105).

Given this situation it is not surprising to find non-physical needs are often somaticised. Take the example of Barbara who was happily married and the mother of one teenage daughter. Barbara had advanced cancer of the ovary and was receiving an opioid for pelvic discomfort. The pain gradually worsened and ultimately she was admitted to the local palliative care unit where the pain was noted to be worse at night, unresponsive to extra doses of medication and frequently accompanied by episodes of panic. The night staff felt this pain had more than a physical cause and encouraged Barbara to talk about her needs and wants. Through tears she spoke about her fear of dying, her concern for her daughter, and of all the things she had hoped to do. The pain settled, the panic attacks resolved and Barbara was discharged home on a smaller rather than a larger dose of opioids.

Steve's story is somewhat similar although his path towards healing was much more complicated and convoluted. He was just 31 when he was admitted to hospital with paraplegia secondary to a rare spinal cord tumour. Steve was a very disturbed young man, having spent most of his life in prison and psychiatric institutions. He was disruptive, controlling, and verbally aggressive, all of which were exacerbated at times of worsening pain. Steve would not talk about his past or the many hurts and regrets that shaped his life. All he wanted was pain relief and a place to smoke. Over the course of several months Steve befriended Mary, an elderly Irish Catholic volunteer and trusted her sufficiently to start journaling his life. Initially this was a liberating experience but as Steve got deeper into his 'pain' he withdrew and put a halt to the journaling exercise. Although he could control the 'external' he was at the mercy of his 'interior' and a nightmare of being chased by a man wanting to kill him with a large knife became a nightly occurrence. These dreams were so disturbing, Steve dreaded sleep and would ask staff to sit with him during the night. In that space he was able to unravel his dream and his life and find meaning in the present experience. His path to healing had just begun but by the time of his death, much of his troubled life and shattered relationships had been reconciled and healed.

IS OUR SYSTEM OF CARE APPROPRIATE FOR THE DYING?

People with a life-threatening illness want to be kept comfortable, to be heard and to lead as normal a life as possible. The same of course is true for everyone but in the case of the former, their shortened life expectancy makes it all the more urgent. The question we need to ask is whether the present system of healthcare facilitates or compromises these goals. Table 2 lists the essential features of the widely practiced biomedical model and the highly regarded but less utilised holistic model. When one looks at the two models it is clear each have their own special role and that one model not only complements but enhances the

TABLE 2. Models of Healthcare

Biomedical	Holistic
Problem orientated	Person orientated
Focus on symptoms and disease	Focus on suffering
Evidence based	Wisdom based
Objective	Subjective
Uni-dimensional	Multi-dimensional
Rational	Intuitive
Jargon	Metaphor
Interventional	Ritualistic
Generic	Individual

other. It is not, therefore, a matter of one or the other but how we can create a framework where the two models are integrated and the goals of comfort and healing co-exist and have equal status.

Recalling the earlier comment of Daniel Callahan, there is an urgent need to address the imbalance in the way care is given. The biomedical model is the dominant paradigm in healthcare and while it serves us well when there is a reasonable chance for cure it leaves much undone when cure is not a reality. The need for holistic care increases not decreases in proportion to the amount of biomedical care given or required (Cassell, 1999) and ultimately there comes a time when the need to prepare for death assumes greater importance than futile attempts to preserve or prolong life.

An integrated model of care exists in principal within palliative care but even there, the danger looms that the gold of holistic care may be lost amongst the grit of biomedical care. The palliation of physical symptoms is an absolutely vital part of palliative care but the goal to palliate or make better when applied to the spiritual and existential domains is frequently counter-productive. We are unable to palliate suffering. The difficulty, says Teilhard de Chardin, "lies not in solving the problem but in expressing it." The goal of solving the 'problem' of suffering is a by-product of the biomedical model and more often than not hinders rather than helps the cause. The essence of caring for those who suffer is found in the words of the philosopher cum cartoonist Michael Leunig (1993): "lead us into the darkness that we may find what lies concealed." Michael Kearney expresses similar sentiments in his book *Mortally Wounded*.

How then do we hospice an old paradigm that fails to adequately address the issue of suffering in those who are dying? This is the question posed by Ken Wilber in his introduction to the book *Consciousness and Healing* (Schlitz et al., 2005). There is of course no easy answer but if one agrees with the essentials of holistic care (Table 3), what is required is a change in the attitude of individual practitioners and in the mindset of institutions. It is a matter of physician heal thyself or in the words of a dying patient, " . . . most important, I found that those around me who were not busy running from their fears could be my closest and only effective friends as death came near" (Kavanaugh, 1974, p. 57). While this statement was made in reference to family and friends, it is equally applicable to those entrusted with the care of the dying.

I recently completed a six month clinical pastoral education attachment in a large teaching hospital. Up until that time I believed I had, as a palliative care doctor, effectively integrated the biomedical and holistic

TABLE 3. Essential Elements of Holistic Care

Ensure physical comfort
Be fully present, authentic, and congruent
Listen
Reflect feelings
Abandon roles and agendas
Suspend judgement, opinions, and beliefs
Take cues from the person
Respect silence
Be aware of own helplessness and vulnerability

models into my clinical practice. Not so. Without recourse to my medical bag of jargon, drugs, and tests and reliant more on interpersonal skills, I found myself struggling to be there when patients talked of their pain and suffering. I was uncomfortable with their vulnerability and helplessness and even more so with my own. Instead of listening I became engrossed with my pain and what I could say to make this better. My agenda to heal got in the way of healing just as it did in my traditional doctor role where I would also try to make 'things' better by withdrawing personally and professionally to the safety of the biomedical model.

Some doctors argue a physician's role is that of a physician and to venture into the sacred and specialized territory of suffering is outside of their brief and not what their patients expect of them. Not all patients agree with this. Anatole Broyard, writing about his experience of being a patient, says of his doctor, "I wish he would give me his whole mind just once, be bonded with me for a brief space, survey my soul as well as my flesh, to get at my illness, for each man is ill in his own way" (Broyard, 1992). Patients want their physicians to be competent but they need them to be caring, as what we ultimately have to offer says Tom Kitwood, "is not technical expertise but ordinary faculties raised to a higher level" (Kitwood, 1997).

CONCLUSION

The pain associated with dying is unique to each and every individual. Finding the right words, symbols, or metaphors to describe their pain is one of many challenges that confront those who are dying. Establishing a link between head and heart helps the dying person come to some understanding about what they feel and this is a fundamental step in their healing process. Opportunities for such dialogue are limited within a problem orientated system of healthcare. Until suffering is seen as something to be heard rather than a problem to be solved, the pain people feel as they die may never see the light of day.

REFERENCES

Ariès, P. (1981). *The hour of our death*. Middlesex: Penguin.

Barker, P. (2000).Working with the metaphor of life and death. *Journal of Medical Ethics: Medical Humanities, 26*, 97-102.

Barker, P. (1999). *The philosophy and practice of psychiatric nursing*. Edinburgh: Churchill Livingstone.

Broyard, A. (1992). *Intoxicated by my illness*. New York: Ballantine Books.

Callahan. D. (1993). Pursuing a peaceful death. *Hastings Centre Report, 23, 4*, 33-38.

Cassell. E. (1982). The nature of suffering and the goals of medicine. *New England Journal of Medicine, 306*, 639-45.

Cassell. E. (1999). Diagnosing suffering: A perspective. *Annals of Internal Medicine, 131*, 531-4.

Cooney, J., & Burton, K. (1986). *Photolanguage Australia*. Catholic Education Office, Sydney, Australia.

Eliot, T. S. (1965). *Murder in the cathedral*. London: Faber and Faber.

Gibran, K. (1979). *The prophet*. London: Heinemann.

Jones, G. (1988). *Magnanimous despair*. Mt. Nebo, Qld: Boombana.

Kavanaugh, R. (1974). *Facing death*. Baltimore: Penguin.

Kearney, M. (1996). *Mortally wounded*. Dublin: Marino Books.

Kitwood, T. (1997). *Dementia reconsidered: The person comes first*. Buckingham: Open University Press.

Leunig, M. (1993). *Common Prayer Collection*. Blackburn: Collins Dove.

Moadel, A., Morgan, C., Fatone, A., Greenan, J., Carter, J., Laruffa, G., Skummy, A., & Dutcher, J. (1999). Seeking meaning and hope: Self-reported spiritual and existential needs among an ethnically-diverse cancer patient population. *Psycho-oncology, 8, 5*, 378-85.

Moore, T. (2004). *Dark Nights of the Soul*. New York: Gotham Books.

Portenoy, R. K., Thaler, H. T., Kornblith, A. B., Lepore, J. M., Friedlander-Klar, H. Coyle, N., Smart-Curley, T., Kemeny, N., Norton, L., Hoskins, W. et al. (1994). Symptom prevalence, characteristics, and distress in a cancer population. *Quality of Life Research, 3, 3*, 183-189.

Saunders, C. (1988). Spiritual Pain. *Journal of Palliative Care, 4, 3*, 29-32.

Schlitz, M., Amorok, T., & Micozzi, M. S. (2005). *Consciousness and healing*. St Louis: Elsevier.

Strang, P., Strang, S., Hultborn, R., & Arner, S. (2004). Existential pain–An entity, a provocation, or a challenge. *Journal of Pain Symptom Management, 27, 3*, 241-50.

Thoreau, H. (1966). *Walden*. New York: The Peter Pauper Press.

Wilber, K. (1991). *Grace and Grit*. Boston: Shambala.

Suffering–
At the Bedside of the Dying

David Currow, MPH, FRACP
Meg Hegarty, RN, BN, MPHC (Pall Care)

SUMMARY. Care of people at the end of life is a challenge for the person with a life-limiting illness, their family and friends, and their professional carers. Clinicians, including pastoral care workers, nurses, doctors, and allied health professionals, find themselves at the bedside of the dying. At times, the professional's sense of self is challenged both by the suffering that they witness (physical, emotional, existential, social, sexual, or financial) and a sense of helplessness to relieve not only the patient's suffering but also that of the people to whom the dying person is close. What framework can help us to deal with the suffering that we cannot help but encounter? Ultimately people connecting in a real and meaningful way with other people is probably the only way that each of us can confront suffering and not have it destroy us. Creating an environment where people can begin to, or continue to connect with others at a level that is mean-

David Currow, MPH, FRACP, is Professor, Department of Palliative and Supportive Services, Flinders University, Adelaide, Australia and Director, Southern Adelaide Palliative Services, Daw Park, Adelaide, Australia (E-mail: david.currow@rgh.sa.gov.au).

Meg Hegarty, RN, BN, MPHC (Pall Care), is affiliated with the Department of Palliative and Supportive Services, Flinders University, Adelaide, Australia (E-mail: meg.hegarty@flinders.edu.au).

[Haworth co-indexing entry note]: "Suffering–At the Bedside of the Dying." Currow, David, and Meg Hegarty. Co-published simultaneously in *Journal of Religion, Spirituality & Aging* (The Haworth Pastoral Press, an imprint of The Haworth Press, Inc.) Vol. 18, No. 2/3, 2006, pp. 123-136; and: *Aging, Spirituality and Palliative Care* (ed: Elizabeth MacKinlay) The Haworth Pastoral Press, an imprint of The Haworth Press, Inc., 2006, pp. 123-136. Single or multiple copies of this article are available for a fee from The Haworth Document Delivery Service [1-800-HAWORTH, 9:00 a.m. - 5:00 p.m. (EST). E-mail address: docdelivery@haworthpress.com].

doi:10.1300/J078v18n02_10

123

ingful for all concerned is a pivotal starting point in dealing with suffering in any encounter with people at the bedside. *[Article copies available for a fee from The Haworth Document Delivery Service: 1-800-HAWORTH. E-mail address: <docdelivery@haworthpress.com> Website: <http://www.HaworthPress.com> © 2006 by The Haworth Press, Inc. All rights reserved.]*

KEYWORDS. Suffering, health care professionals, pastoral care workers, caregivers, end-of-life care, palliative care

To talk about death and dying makes us intolerably anxious . . . about our own eventual fate (and) the pointlessness of our own present lives.

Robert Dessaix (1996, p. 111)

INTRODUCTION

In any clinical practice we are confronted with an enormous amount of suffering. The term suffering is not being used interchangeably with pain nor with grief and bereavement, but as a distinct and separate entity which is independent of, but related to so much of what defines each of us. In caring for people at the end of life, this suffering can be, at times, a major source of ongoing distress despite optimal physical symptom control.

Suffering is something with which each of us personally continues to struggle and on which none of us is expert. Suffering can challenge our world view and our belief systems. We see significant suffering both in clinical practice and in the world around us. How we deal with suffering as humans and as health and pastoral care professionals continues to be an almost unfathomable problem. This paper, more than anything, reflects on this struggle.

At the centre of this challenge is the contrast between what each of us believe we would do if faced with a life-limiting illness and the reality for most people in this circumstance. The diagnosis of a life-limiting illness (such as cancer, AIDS, end-stage organ failure, or motor neurone disease) is a time of challenge and of reflection, of often rapidly re-prioritising life (not expecting to see your next birthday allows intense focus on what is really important in life) and allowing time for things that may not have had enough attention. Dramatic life changes, such as global travel or skydiving are rare (although jumping out of a perfectly good plane at 10,000 feet is perhaps a powerful metaphor for the unknown of both the process of dying and of death itself). Instead, people mostly focus on relationships, reducing study and work commitments, refining life goals, exploring their own relationship with the universe, and restructuring finances (Steinhauser, 2000). Physically for most people, this is a time of life not filled with energy, but a time of reflection and diminishing physical reserves.

For many people actually facing the spectre of a progressive life-limiting illness, the song "Ol' Man River" captures their response in a much more realistic way: " . . . tired of living, scared of dying. . . . "

Emotionally and physically, there is the challenge of how we as clinicians and caregivers best support people who face death as an expected outcome of their current illness. Opportunities to support these people should be a major focus for health providers and for our system of social support, given that approximately half of all deaths in developed countries would be considered 'expected deaths.'

There are three key areas that will be explored in this article. How we characterise suffering is a key concern as we try to understand suffering. Who suffers with people in the setting of a life-limiting illness? Finally, how can we each respond to suffering?

CHARACTERISING SUFFERING

Suffering is, in many ways, a mystery. Attempting to characterise suffering is an important step in our attempts to understand it. Personal, cultural and social components will have an impact on the way each of us suffers. While many aspects of the experiences of suffering can be understood, its very presence challenges notions of a benevolent human existence. The struggle to understand suffering has engaged people since earliest times. Poets and artists have expressed this since the paintings on cave walls (Heyse-Moore, 1996). The major world religions have generated constructs that seek to explain in some way or give meaning to the whole human experience including suffering. These writings have also given us rich metaphors of our struggle with the problem of suffering. Universally expressed existential questions cannot be adequately met without a struggle of the spirit (Chittister, 2003).

Response to suffering can span the spectrum from enhanced compassion, understanding, and strengthened resilience through to fear, avoidance, and a lowered threshold for any future suffering.

Ultimately, suffering is something which is intensely personal. It is as subjective as pain or shortness of breath. Two people with *apparently* identical challenges may have totally different perceptions of their suffering. One may rate herself as having no suffering and the other may rate herself as experiencing uncontrolled and overwhelming suffering. There is no objective measure of the degree of suffering and as a result, we are challenged by the fact that we cannot see what this looks like for another person.

Suffering is Subjective

Suffering is a unique entity which may be independent of the obvious factors that may contribute to it. One cannot *"anticipate what she describes as her source of suffering"* as Eric Cassell points out in reflecting on a young woman's breast cancer (Cassell, 1983, p. 522). There were the physical aspects of her suffering (physical deformity, the side-effects of treatment that left her body scarred and damaged), her social suffering ('the isolation and social death' experienced long before physical death as some family and friends withdraw), the suffering of her self-image and the existential suffering of impending death that she was experiencing. As a distinct and independent entity, we cannot simply relate it to what we as health professionals or fellow humans see in the clinical encounter. This subjectivity also contributes to the isolation that is engendered for many as they suffer. The ensuing strain on relationships may test even the strongest and most committed relationship. Such strain is further challenged by changes in roles and locus of control in almost all relationships. Suffering is something with which many people grapple, attempting to work through it.

In science, we seek cause-and-effect relationships. We seek such relationships to explain the world in which we live and our responses to this world. How often have we sat at the bedside with someone agonizingly looking for the cause of what is happening to them–"Why me?" "Why now in my life?" or "What could I possibly have done to deserve this?" The ultimate product of this search can be itself a source of suffering. An absence of a causal relationship further challenges many people in these circumstances. Depending on one's world view, the soul-searching and (potential) guilt of "I must have done something really bad to be faced with this illness" takes a great deal of time and energy for many people to reconcile at the end of life. An apparently rational approach to this question fails to provide answers or, at times, solace.

Suffering Is Context and Culturally Specific

At another level, is suffering in part explained by a dissonance between our expectations and the reality we are or shall experience? A young man in the highlands of New Guinea brought his wife to the hospital close to death. She died a few hours after arriving at hospital from an illness, which in a developed country:

a. would not occur, or
b. if it did occur, would have been diagnosed earlier and would have been easily treated.

She died and while her body was still warm he came into the ward, gently covered her head with a sheet and walked out of the hospital. He was starting a 40 mile walk home. One of the hospital staff walked with him for a way. He made it clear that he had to go back to his village because he had four young children to feed and a garden to tend to. Without the garden they would all starve. This did not mean that he was not suffering, but the context in which he had lived all his life had generated very different constructs for his day-to-day life. For him, his expectation was of a . . . life-death-life-death . . . cycle where death was as much a certainty as life itself. For those of us who live in a society that allows us to exist with clear, long-term plans stretching well into the future, we may be faced with very different types of suffering from people who subsist. The pressures and tensions that underlie suffering may be defined by societal norms that do not translate easily between cultures.

Indigenous people around the world, whether in Canada, the highlands of Vietnam, east Malaysia, the Maori or Aboriginal and Torres Strait Islanders in Australia, have a history of disempowerment, being disenfranchised and experiencing cultural destruction either through systematic processes, inadvertent actions or both. Such suffering is not lost quickly and its echoes are felt through generations to come.

Threatened Personhood

Inherent in the news that someone has a life-limiting illness is a threat to self, to one's very existence. This alone is a significant cause of suffering for many people. This is not simply about separation from people who are close to them, 'symptom control' nor potential future loss of independence. It is that one's current existence as we know it ceases. In response to this challenge, different people will react differently. Supporting people through their responses to a limited life-expectancy is a central responsibility of all carers for people at the end-of-life.

Perhaps more poignantly, Cassell characterises suffering as a "threat to self" or a "threat to a sense of self" (Cassell, 1983). This gives far broader definition to all that suffering can encapsulate. If it is a threat to our personhood then a wide range of insults can influence this. It is not just our physical wellbeing but our social, sexual, emotional, financial, or spiritual sense of wellbeing that can contribute to and, at times, drive suffering.

Corporate Suffering

Why did pubs in Republican Ireland close for Princess Diana's funeral? Why were you unable to buy a flower in Northern Europe in the days leading up to that funeral? Why did 2.5 billion people stop for an hour to watch a funeral for someone they had never met and whose direct impact on their lives was at best for many the fantasy of a princess who died a violent death? What of the response to a Pope dying at the age of 84, yet the world stopped? Is there a case that we, as a community, have tried so hard to insulate ourselves from suffering that we need to seek an opportunity for a communal response to suffering in such circumstances? Is it that we have tried so hard to avoid an opportunity to address the challenge of suffering that we need a communal (and safer) place to explore these questions? Do these outpourings of grief illustrate an unmet need for connection to our fellow human beings at a time when our mortality is so clearly challenged and where rites and rituals help us deal with the situation?

Anticipatory Suffering

The other phenomenon for us is anticipatory suffering. Given full knowledge and our ability, particularly in the Western world, to plan our life ahead in weeks, months, years, or decades, we have the fear of what life will one day hold. Many people's ability to live 'in the moment' is severely limited. Our fear of one day requiring physical care is a common concern when people are faced with significant illness (Steinhauser, 2000).

Is Suffering 'Self-Levelling'?

Health related quality of life is framed by the absence of problems or a deficit of negatives. By contrast, quality of life in a psychological construct is about subjective well-being. Even in the face of significant physical symptoms or psychiatric problems, subjective wellbeing can be surprisingly well preserved for many people. People who lose mobility and become either paraplegic or quadriplegic through trauma may have a significant decrease in subjective quality of life for a time. However, health related quality of life is likely to improve significantly as time passes (Damschroder, 2005; Dowler, 2001). Is suffering a specific subjective sensation that directly impairs global quality of life, lying on a continuum with other psychological factors that ultimately determine our sense of wellbeing?

Bob Cummins and his group are exploring the concept that quality of life in its broadest subjective sense may well be self-levelling (Cummins, 2005). That is to say, quality of life returns to a person's own normative point after any change in circumstances (good or bad), independent of the narrow confines of physical health. Further, issues of quality of life are defined predominately by a sense of well-being largely driven by the relationships that we enjoy. These same relationships are themselves often altered irrevocably at the time of people being diagnosed with a life-limiting illness. A continuing tension for many people is how to break the news to other people that they have a life-limiting illness or, as a member of that person's family or as a friend, how best to respond. Despite increases in suffering at times, do our coping mechanisms return to our own individual norm?

Is There a 'Suffering Quotient'?

Is suffering limited for each of us at any given time in this same normative process? Many decades ago, C. Northcote Parkinson defined Parkinson's Law–'that work expands to fill the time available' (Parkinson, 1957). It may be that for many of us, suffering also fills the available space in our life, creating for each of us a normative level of suffering. It may be that there is a suffering quotient for each person and that regardless of the life circumstances (excellent life circumstance through to dire distress and real and present danger), each of us can only deal within a self-defined range of suffering. This range may be influenced by both corporate norms (culture, religious beliefs, and societal expectations) and individual factors such as personality (do we see the world as a glass half full or a glass half empty?). At one end of this spectrum even if the suffering is not apparent from our life circumstances, we are capable of creating enough suffering to fill that space. The person with no financial worries and good physical health may still perceive themselves to be suffering from challenges which in other more pressing circumstances may seem trivial. For such a person, Parkinson's Law defines almost perfectly what is happening.

At the other end of the spectrum, any objective measure would suggest, for much of the world's population, that the suffering they experience daily would be enough to totally overwhelm anyone not used to such circumstances. We are able to block some aspects of suffering, rationalise others and live on despite dire circumstances that could otherwise destroy us.

Like pain, the degree of suffering may not seem congruent at times with the expression of that suffering. Some people seem to take great suffering in stride; for others, seemingly small perturbations lead to an overwhelming sense of suffering.

WHO SUFFERS AT THE END OF LIFE?

During the consultation in which it was confirmed that Robert Dessaix was diagnosed as being HIV positive (before the advent of triple therapy), he describes in vivid detail his feeling of 'sliding downwards into blackness . . . already in another world' (Dessaix, 1996). Receiving and dealing with that news and its consequences reverberate instantly through many lives. Having insight into future health states and their detailed consequences must influence our response to news such as the diagnosis of cancer, HIV, or end-stage organ failure. The ability to know the future in detail is an expectation for being a fully informed consumer but, like everything else, this may have a downside for many people.

The person with a life-limiting illness may suffer. The physical suffering at the end of life is real, and although there is much we can do to ameliorate the physical symptoms across many life-limiting illnesses, physical suffering may still be present. In addition, existential suffering raises questions of why we are here, what does life mean and what are the legacies that will characterise life? These are difficult questions for many people and create anxiety and concerns. Social suffering is yet another component of suffering often reflected on by people at the end of life. People describe social death long before their physical death, as friends and families, not knowing what to say or do in these circum-stances, simply cease to have contact. This social suffering impacts on the sense of self in terms of roles and relationships with others and hence the context in which many of us live and experience ourselves. Is this 'aloneness' because at a community level we fear to share our own feelings of inadequacy and helplessness, and so fail to reach out to the person who is so alone?

In clinical practice, there are two profoundly lonely places that one finds oneself. The first is the person whose entire spiritual life with a history of strongly held religious beliefs, finds that belief is failing or has failed them. A woman for whom we cared had what she character-ised as a strong religious belief. For her there was a 'cop' in the sky who ensured that good people had good things happen to them and bad peo-ple had bad things happen to them. Her illness was considered by her a 'bad thing' and yet she could identify nothing that she had done which should cause it. This shattered her belief system and left her unable to talk to her family or her religious mentors about it. Further, she was afraid to be angry with the god in whom she no longer believed, and a day from death was in a lonely and desolate place. There was no time to explore or redefine a more realistic view of her god in her world, a pro-cess which would demand openness, time, and a willingness to confront the ambiguity and paradoxes of reality challenging her belief system. Living with the uncertainty of a changing belief system can be both painful and, for some, a time of enormous personal growth.

The second lonely place for fellow humans, especially clinicians, is where a person, in the absence of depression, can identify no reason to live and is totally unconnected to anyone else in the world. Some people in this circumstance can identify no other person with whom they have ever felt a connection. Is this an ultimate form of suffering and, if so, how do we support someone in such a position? For people who are ac-tively suffering, we have all seen peers and colleagues who have tried to create a framework for the person to deal with their suffering. As one of the most intensely personal sensations, the answers for suffering come from the person themselves, in the context of their life, their relation-ships, and their belief system. The presence and strength of other hu-mans in times of such loneliness is important, if only to 'borrow' communal hope or share experiences of transcendence. At our peril, we, as health professionals, try to create a framework for other people to deal with suffering. We, time and again, at the end of life see people move from a situation where life is bearable to a situation where aspects of life are becoming unbearable.

Caregiver Suffering

Caregivers are challenged by their own suffering at the end of the life of someone that they care for (Hinds, 1992). One source of such suffering is the person who at the bedside of the person with the life-limiting illness feels helpless to 'fix' things. Our helplessness to make things right and that feeling of impotence that ensues is a source of great suffering for caregivers both while they are in the role and as they later reflect back on their roles. Caregivers are also asked to take on roles for which they are ill prepared. For the 'baby boomer generation,' many spouses are caring for someone for the first time in their life and then watching, again for the first time in their lives, that person die in their fifth or sixth decades. Their grandparents died when they were young. Their parents and siblings are all well and alive as are their children.

As 'Generation X' ages, we are going to run out of caregivers and the demands on those caregivers who will be available is likely to heighten caregiver suffering. Whose suffering in this circumstance takes precedence–the patient's or the caregiver's? How is the cumulative suffering of repeated loss dealt with? What outcomes are compromised as we try to deal with everyone's suffering?

Family Suffering

There is also family suffering. This is particularly reflected in communication breakdown, a sense of lack of support and the enormous lifestyle disruption that occurs in people at the end of life. This should not be underestimated as we look at the work of David Kissane in family functioning styles at the end of life (Kissane, 2003).

Health Professionals' Suffering

Most health professionals come to their clinical roles in order to make things right, fix things, or to cure. Repeated confrontations with mortality may well have an enormous impact on how we as health professionals see our roles both professionally and more broadly, how we define ourselves away from work. If our 'sense of self' is strongly defined by our professional roles, then a sense of inadequacy and hence a threat to our sense of self may be the consequence of repeated exposure to death. After all, death for many clinicians is firstly perceived as a 'failure' until proven otherwise, rather than as a consequence of living. There was a moving account in the British Medical Journal soon after

the Hillsborough soccer disaster (Heller, 1989). The first general practitioner on the site reflected on his helplessness and the total inadequacy that he felt both in the role and on later reflecting on his role.
Although there was an overwhelming camaraderie of the people who
worked under the grandstand that afternoon, there was also a sense of
enormous loss and the fact that life would never be the same for them
again despite the excellence of their training. The way in which this
doctor had his sense of self threatened personally and professionally is
a poignant statement.

HOW THEN DO WE APPROACH SUFFERING?

Within the professional context, Balfour Mount is quoted as saying
that suffering is a profound awareness of personal vulnerability. This
probably related well to Henri Nouwen's concept of the 'wounded
healer' (Nouwen, 1979). C.S. Lewis is quoted as saying that he spent so
much time avoiding suffering that he was unable to fully appreciate delight (Lewis, 1998). The full impact of this last comment bears thinking
about. Although delight may be an antonym of suffering, it is not, of itself, an answer to it. What is the answer to it? We have all read Viktor
Frankl (Frankl, 1986). Although as a result of suffering, people may
find meaning, this in no way suggests that suffering is of itself good.
The fact that people, after horrific suffering, can find 'good' is a testament to the human spirit and not a reflection on the value of suffering. It
again highlights how people can reconcile and grow through the enormous paradoxes encountered in life.

Eric Cassell, early in his writing on suffering, suggested that resilience may be part of the response to suffering. People have different
mechanisms and levels of resilience in different circumstances. Later,
Cassell, with something that may be interpreted as nihilism, stresses
that suffering is just part of the human condition. This statement simply
states the case that suffering "is" without any value judgement (Cassell,
1991). Avoidable suffering should be avoided. Unavoidable suffering
should be met with the tools which we, individually and communally,
have developed to deal with such challenges in life.

Is it healing–moving towards wholeness (emotional, social, existential, spiritual) with the honesty and intensity of that struggle–that is the
antidote to suffering? One may see suffering (a threat to one's sense of
self) as being at the opposite extreme of a continuum with healing
(achieving wholeness). Exploring such a relationship suggests that suf-

fering is in its strictest sense being less than whole, and most of us therefore suffer in our lives.

If suffering is a sense of self that is damaged, threatened or otherwise compromised, then perhaps the reality is that the solution to suffering is connectedness–to ourselves, to others, to our sense of God or life. As health professionals, even in the midst of suffering we are not asked to find solutions as much as to be there for that person in a very present and tangible way. This is something which is not innate but can be learned by health professionals and by others so that people are not abandoned. Creating the connectedness may well be at the heart of supporting someone who is suffering. It is not a clever set of preconceived constructs that give suffering meaning, but of a person connecting with another person, in whatever circumstances they find themselves. Recognising our interconnectedness as humans on a joint journey through life is a crucial first step in this process.

A CONNECTED RESPONSE

This recognition of shared humanity is a transformative experience for both carer and the one cared for (Bambery, 1997). It invites a relationship in which the carer's presence is one of humility, honesty, openness, and trust, creating a relationship of mutuality and respect for the *wisdom within the suffering person's spirit* (Hegarty, 2001b). Such presence creates a safe space within which the person who suffers "is supported in expressing and exploring the anguish, the paradoxes and the wisdom in the inner darkness, the deep questions with no easy answers, the interplay of hope, fear, denial, and acceptance (Hegarty, 2001a, p. 4).

For some, the exploration of the meaning of their suffering leads to a transcendence of the suffering–not an escape, but working towards a sense of peace and hope. For others, the suffering remains with no consolation.

Being with someone who suffers and recognizing our own limits is for most of us the most difficult and challenging thing we are called to do (Cassidy, 1988). At very deep levels, real connection with a suffering person evokes in us *the fear of our own undoing* (Barnard, 1995). It challenges us with intimations of our own vulnerability and mortality. It requires an ability to let go of the need to have answers and to not abandon the suffering person. Paradoxically, the darkness of shared struggle with suffering and the letting go of illusions of invincibility can be graced gifts–insights leading to growth and openness to experiences of healing, acceptance and love for our wounded, vulnerable selves. Suffering and hope can be experiences that are simultaneous and in no way are contradictory. It is in the wrestling with suffering that growth towards hope often happens.

CONCLUSION

Suffering occurs in many guises. It is a subjective experience, differing for each of us. Our responses to suffering and our capacity to deal with it vary widely. As clinicians and carers, our own and others' suffering affects us deeply. Yet within the mystery of suffering there remain unanswered questions. Despite all of these factors, suffering is a human universal and it seems that our shared humanness is healing in times of suffering.

We forget that when John Donne wrote "No man is an island, entire of itself " that the next line was "Any man's death diminishes me, because I am involved in Mankind." This connectedness is the one way that suffering–physical, emotional, social, sexual, spiritual, existential–can be addressed. As a distinct entity, suffering needs to be recognised and addressed. As a subjective entity we need to explore with that person *their* suffering in the context of *their* life, all of *their* life experience, the 'baggage' they bring to this moment in life and their future expectations in order to understand both the suffering now and the (anticipatory) suffering that they may face in the future. We also need the courage to recognise our own response to suffering as we sit at the bedside.

REFERENCES

Bambery, J. K. (1997). Spirituality as a healing force. In S. Ronaldson (Ed.), *Spirituality: The heart of nursing*. Melbourne: Ausmed Publications.

Barnard, D. (1995). The promise of intimacy and the fear of our own undoing. *Journal of Palliative Care, 11*, 22-26.

Cassell, E. J. (1983). The relief of suffering. *Archives of Internal Medicine, 143*, 522-3.

Cassell, E. J. (1991). *Recognizing suffering. Hastings Center Report, 21, 3*, 24-31.

Cassidy, S. (1988). *Sharing the darkness: The spirituality of caring*. Darton: Longman & Todd.

Chittister, J. (2003). *Scarred by struggle, transformed by hope*. Grand Rapids, MI: William B. Eerdmans Publishing Company.

Cummins, R. (2005). *In supportive care of the urology patient.* Oxford: Oxford University Press.

Damschroder, L. J., Zikmund-Fisher, B. J., & Ubel, P. A. (2005). The impact of considering adaptation in health state valuation. *Social Science Medicine, 61,* 267-277.

Dessaix, R. (1996). *Night letters.* Melbourne: Macmillan Publishing.

Donne, J. (1572-1631). In 'Devotions Upon Emergent Occasions' Meditation XVII 'Now, this bell tolling softly.'

Dowler, R., Richards, J. S., Putzke, J. D., Gordon, W., & Tate, D. (2001). Impact of demographic and medical factors on satisfaction with life after a spinal cord injury: A normative study. *Journal Spinal Cord Medicine, 24,* 87-91.

Frankl, V. (1986). *The doctor and the soul.* New York, NY: Random House–Vintage Books Edition.

Hegarty, M. (2001a). Strangers in a Wild Place. Compass a: 3-7.

Hegarty, M. (2001b). The dynamic of hope: Hoping in the face of death. *Progress in Palliative Care, 9,* 42-47.

Heller, T. (1989). Personal and medical memories from Hillsborough. *British Medical Journal, 299,* 1596-1598.

Heyse-Moore, L. H. (1996). On spiritual pain in the dying. *Mortality, 1,* 297-315.

Hinds, C. (1992). Suffering: A relatively unexplored phenomenon among family caregivers of non-institutionalized patients with cancer. *Journal of Advanced Nursing, 17, 8,* 918-25.

Kissane, D. W., McKenzie, M., McKenzie, D. P., Forbes, A., O'Neill, I., & Bloch, S. (2003). Psychosocial morbidity associated with patterns of family functioning in palliative care: Baseline data from the Family Focused Grief Therapy controlled trial. *Palliative Medicine, 17,* 527-537.

Lewis, C. S. (1998). *Surprised by joy.* London: Harper Collins Religious.

Nouwen, H. (1979). *The wounded healer.* New York, NY: Doubleday.

Parkinson, C. N. (1957). *Parkinson's law.* London: Houghton Miffin.

Steinhuaser, K. E., Christakis, N. A., Clipp, E. C., McNeilly, M., McIntyre, L., & Tulsky, J. A. (2000). Factors considered important at the end of life by patients, families, physicians, and other care providers. *Journal of the American Medical Association, 284,* 2476-2482.

Joy in the Midst of Suffering: Clowning as Care of the Spirit in Palliative Care

Jenny Thompson-Richards, BA, BSoc Admin, MSW

SUMMARY. We find joy in the midst of suffering at Daw House, a palliative care unit. Stories, ranging from moments of gentle tenderness to wild hilarity, speak of profound joy and of the courage of those who participate. We articulate some of the *why* and *how* of caring clowning. Clown Doctors aim to affirm people as people with richly storied lives, to give permission for both laughter and tears, and to bring consolation to the spirit. The art of clowning means that we seek to elevate people, to sensitively tailor music, touch, and colour to the interests of those we encounter, to invite a sense of wonder and spontaneity and to work to transform situations through the imagination. *[Article copies available for a fee from The Haworth Document Delivery Service: 1-800-HAWORTH. E-mail address: <docdelivery@haworthpress.com> Website: <http://www.HaworthPress.com> © 2006 by The Haworth Press, Inc. All rights reserved.]*

Jenny Thompson-Richards, BA, BSoc Admin, MSW, is Member, AASW, and The Humour Foundation, and Social Worker, Southern Adelaide Palliative Services, Daw Park Adelaide, Australia (Web-site: www.clowndoctors.com.au).

The author thanks the many people who allowed her into their lives and to Ann Harrington for manuscript help. The author also thanks her fellow silly people: David Cronin, a.k.a. Dr. Heebie Jeebie, Dianne Bodein Walters, a.k.a. Dr. TeapoT, and the Humour Foundation for their generous support.

[Haworth co-indexing entry note]: "Joy in the Midst of Suffering: Clowning as Care of the Spirit in Palliative Care." Thompson-Richards, Jenny. Co-published simultaneously in *Journal of Religion, Spirituality & Aging* (The Haworth Pastoral Press, an imprint of The Haworth Press, Inc.) Vol. 18, No. 2/3, 2006, pp. 137-152; and: *Aging, Spirituality and Palliative Care* (ed: Elizabeth MacKinley) The Haworth Pastoral Press, an imprint of The Haworth Press, Inc., 2006, pp. 137-152. Single or multiple copies of this article are available for a fee from The Haworth Document Delivery Service [1-800-HAWORTH, 9:00 a.m. - 5:00 p.m. (EST). E-mail address: docdelivery@haworthpress.com].

KEYWORDS. Joy, suffering, transcendence, affirmation, spirituality, playfulness

THE WORK

Three Clown Doctors, Dr. Heebie Jeebie, Dr. TeapoT, and Dr. Wooops (myself), have visited Daw House weekly for almost four years. We are part of the Humour Foundation, a charity that has over forty Clown Doctors in Australia. Clowns bring their own character and skills. Dr. Heebie Jeebie dresses smartly in a red and white striped shirt. He does magic and improvises with music on a yellow ukulele, harmonica, and with coloured hand bells. Dr. TeapoT wears a green tea cosy on her head out of which protrudes blonde hair teased into a handle and spout. She offers many varieties of "tea." Dr. Wooops delights in clumsy dancing, rainbow colours, and *cat scans*–shoulder massages from Dr. Cat, a wooden massager. We exaggerate our own foibles. In everyday life I mix my words, so Wooops embellishes this weakness to create impossible medical word salads. We perform in pairs. Daw House is a stately, homely former residence set amidst lovely gardens. It accommodates fifteen people who are admitted for a variety of reasons–respite, symptom management, or because they are dying.

Our protocol means that we:

- Carefully observe infection control procedures;
- Seek a briefing from the nursing staff and record our interactions;
- Give precedence to clinical procedures, but we are willing to stay if our presence helps;
- Always seek the patient's permission (verbally or non-verbally) to enter a room.

Dianne Bodein Walters, a.k.a. Dr. TeapoT, once described us as *"purveyors of joy."* Joy is not an isolated, abstract concept, a commodity that we give to others, but it springs out of relationships. Our job is to foster a warm, light-hearted atmosphere that evokes joy. Joy is quite different from happiness. Happiness depends on pleasure, and good circumstances. Joy is much more profound and encompasses a sense of contentment in all circumstances. Joy embraces a deep, quiet peace and an exuberance that bubbles over. The *why* and *how* of clowning in a palliative care unit relates closely to finding joy in the midst of grief. We evoke playfulness, invite a sense of wonder and treasure the smallest responses. Stories from our work are the best way to illustrate this theme. All names are changed and I have annotated each story in italics to explain our thoughts and reflections.

CLOWN DOCTORS SEEK TO AFFIRM PEOPLE AS PEOPLE WITH RICHLY STORIED LIVES

We Seek to Affirm People as People Before Role, Diagnosis, or Status

Daw House has a large open day room and after our briefing we often begin there. We happily interact with anyone–patients, volunteers, orderlies, nurses, doctors, and visitors alike. We offer shoulder and head massages and camaraderie. We gladly oblige when staff call out "Hey, what about my massage?" Often it gives people new to Daw House an opportunity to observe and see what we are about.

We Seek to Draw Out the Other Threads of People's Richly Storied Lives

Illness is one thread of someone's life story but only one thread. We seek to elicit dignifying threads of people's life stories. These threads can be of any nature. We notice something in the room, family photos, flowers, or a conversation topic and this allows us to explore, to engage, and to build play around those interests. I relate this story because it reflects a regular feature of our work.

A family welcomes us into the room and we meet Paul who is very weak. Anne, his wife and Jill, his daughter sit nearby. In the midst of massages and friendly repartee something prompts Heebie Jeebie to sing "Somewhere over the rainbow." Anne and Jill join in too. We all forget the words at one point and Paul's thin voice finishes the line. We "ooh and ahh." This prompts Ann and Jill to enthusiastically discuss how Paul had the best recall of lyrics in the family. Ann laughs and tells how she would lose track of him whilst shopping. She would find him helping elderly people to reach high shelves or opening doors. As we leave, Paul is smiling while Ann and Jill continue to discuss his many endearing qualities.

They are celebrating the many richly interwoven threads of Paul's life story. Stories have power to richly enhance lives, transform the way we see and interact with the world and reveal the wonders of the human spirit.

WE GIVE PERMISSION FOR BOTH LAUGHTER AND TEARS

A man visiting his wife when offered a *cat scan* said, "I'd love one but I'd cry."

Another daughter was struggling with grief. TeapoT offered her cup of "*Sereni-Tea*" while Wooops massaged her shoulders and she began to cry.

We recognize that touch, music and TeapoT's teas sometimes evoke sadness.

Many Times Laughter and Tears Intermingle

We met Pat many times. She was always very enthusiastic about everyone despite her significant short-term memory loss. Today we are briefed that she is dying. I see Susan, her daughter, in the day room and offer her a *cat scan*.

"Hey, that's good. He must be a talented cat," says Susan as she turns to show the slogan on her T-shirt–*Behind every gifted woman is a talented cat*. We laugh. I ask if we can see Pat.

"Oh come, she'll love it."

We enter by opening the curtain enough to see Susan and Pam sitting with their mother and the music therapist with her harp. We offer to return later but the music therapist assures that she is finished.

TeapoT asks, "How can we possibly follow that act?"

"We can't. Let's go away and they may forget about her wonderful playing. Bye."

TeapoT says, "Let's celebrate with a song."

She gets out a large, silk, rainbow material, hands one end to Susan, and we all sing '*Somewhere over the rainbow.*' Then TeapoT suggests a tea party since it is Pat's birthday. Pam wants a *cat scan* since she has heard about it from Susan. Wooops engages in lots of banter with an abundance of mishaps with medical terms. We all laugh heartily.

TeapoT gets out her tea cosies. They willingly put them on their heads. Wooops tells Susan that she looks like a bishop. TeapoT puts a pastel crocheted tea cosy on Pat's head. Pam looks very silly in a yellow cotton one. We all guffaw loudly about how ridiculous we look. TeapoT gets out thimble-size, clown teacups and shows them her book of *Dr.*

TeapoT's Famous Medicinal Tea Labels. It has many-coloured draw-ings of each tea: *Naugh-Tea, Frivoli-Tea. . . .* She backs into the corner of the room so we can all see the labels.

Suddenly, Pat snores a little more loudly.

TeapoT quips, "Call that a snore Pat, I can teach you to snore."

From her tiny clown teapot, TeapoT eyes Susan and pours out *Sereni-Tea* for her, and deliberates before giving *Tranquili-Tea* to Pam. Wooops gets *Moosicali-Tea*, greedily and noisily slurps it, realizes her rudeness and apologises loudly. More laughs. TeapoT shows them a beautiful scene with a curving path that curves through green rolling hills and vanishes over the horizon. She pours out *Eterni-Tea* for Pat. We all draw breath. We pause. Susan and Pam have wet eyes. The act of collecting the teacups and tea cosies brings forth more silliness and laughs. We leave with a flourish.

We try to begin and finish with the mood of the room and since they welcomed us enthusiastically, we matched this and entered and exited with energy. We acknowledged Pat throughout. We gave her a tea cosy and a cup of tea. TeapoT brought dignity when she claimed to snore more loudly. Both daughters sighed as they were given their tea, a very common response to receiving Sereni-Tea and Tranquil-Tea. There was a poignant silence when we acknowledged Pat's imminent death with a cup of Eterni-Tea. Later, when I ask Susan's permission to write this story, she confirms that this was the most significant moment. Times of hilarity cradled the potent moment of tears.

WE SEEK TO BRING CONSOLATION TO THE SPIRIT

First, Connecting with People Is Our Highest Priority

Susan is newly transferred from another hospital–huddled up under her bed coverings, facing the window. Her son and daughter, in their early thirties, sit with her. We were playfully singing quietly with her roommate. We work in pairs but Wooops goes over tentatively to intro-duce herself, ready to exit if not wanted. She does a quiet little trip and a "Hullllooo I'm Dr. Wooooops." I got my silly, piggy rubber nose right close to Susan and she met my eyes fully. We smile at each other. Time stands respectfully aside. "Hullo bountiful." I gently *cat scan* her shoul-ders, give one to her children and leave.

She died the next day. They wrote in a card, "Thanks to everyone at Daw House and thanks to Dr. Wooops for the compassion and cheer." The com-

bination of the words "compassion and cheer" seems to capture the heart of our work that is to bring a sense of consolation of the spirit.

We Treasure Small Responses: Laughter Is Not Our Measure of Success

According to Oscar Wilde, "Where there is sorrow there is Holy Ground." Many times we sense that we are invited into holy ground as in the story of John's smile.

I notice two men outside of a room that we had decided against entering. We were briefed that John was dying. As I approach them–one notices the "I is the insultant" badge. They joke about this. Tom, the younger brother, is very tall and keeps his distance.

Colin, the older brother, readily accepts the offer to sit and have a *cat scan* and he talks about his Dad. He becomes very enthusiastic when Wooops brings out the *Bliss Machine* to give him a head massage. Colin eagerly convinces Tom to have one too. After the bliss treatment, Tom tells Colin–"We got to get these guys to see Mum." He comes out after a minute to usher us in. Mavis is sitting there holding John's hand. He looks unconscious. We enter. He opens his eyes and gives a smile. Wooops comes close up and he slowly focuses.

"Hey, he's here!"

The "Ooh and aaahs" from all three are loud and prolonged. He smiles–a wonderfully, gentle, toothless smile. It is clear from the oohs that his alert smile is water in the desert and tears appear in all our eyes.

"Cop that smile" Colin elbows his younger brother.

They smile. "Ooh how precious . . . this is priceless. The smile, the smile!!"

In raspy breath John asks, "What's your name?"

"Wooops" and "Heebie Jeebie"

The priceless smile widens. Heebie gives Mavis a head massage. Wooops shows her the soft brush and she tells John that it is like a soft rabbit and she brushes his arms with it. He closes his eyes and enjoys. Wooops takes his hand and he grasps it strongly. With his other hand he holds onto Colin.

"Wow, you still have got some strength there," says Colin.

We just take time smiling into his eyes. He seems to soak it up. He pulls Wooops towards him. Wooops bends over and gives him a kiss on the cheek. At some point, Tom starts taking photos. John tries to say something. He wants Tom in the photo too.

We all shuffle in and put our heads close in–they want to capture the smile. He is very still except for the grin.

The two sons continue to utter things like–"You've made our day guys."

Heebie plays and we all sing, "When Irish eyes are smiling."

John rasps, "Hey listen."

"We're all listening."

"Not much time left now"

"Not much, no." says Mavis.

He wants another kiss–this time he wants to give the kisses–tender, tiny kisses.

More groans and Tom also kisses his Dad on the head. "Love you Dad."

Mavis says, "You've been blessed, very precious time this."

More photos. Tom says, "We going to get that smile Dad." He rests his eyes but still smiles. Mavis admires Wooop's costume so she shows off her new swirling skirt, does some kicks to Heebie's song and reveals the bloomers underneath. They laugh with tears in their eyes. Wooops gives Mavis a hug.

"I've nursed him all this time until now," and then she whispers "No not long now."

The sons want more photos of us. Wooops says "Gee, are they always this bossy?" Mavis laughs and says, "Yes." Each son gives us big bear hugs with lots of thanks. We all have wet eyes.

His family is obviously very grateful that, after several days of unresponsiveness, John opens his eyes and smiles. Colin described his smile as "water in the desert." We were privileged to be there at the right time. To a casual observer, we did very little, but responded to their wishes. We treasure lovingly held eye contact, a warm touch or slight smile. Naturally, we welcome healthy laugher but it is not our measure of success.

We Seek to Identify with People in Their Vulnerably so That They Can Transcend Their Circumstances

I relate some of our times with Audrey.

Week 1. We put out heads around her room to find Audrey, 70 with a Frank and Norma. We were briefed that her husband had dementia, was in care and that they were childless. Wooops asks, "Hulloooo is it ok to wisit you?" She nods and looks a little perplexed and so with little trip we enter into the room. I show them Dr. Cat, the little wooden black and white massager, and then offer *cat scans*. They all "Ooh and ah ah" with pleasure. They laugh.

Franks asks, "Hey do you play that thing?"

Heebie Jeebie plays and we all readily sing, "You are My Sunshine." Wooops proudly does her simpleton's dance, one leg stuck in the air at a time.

Week 2. We have a fun time with Audrey and her visitors. This time Frank tells lots of jokes, and at one point hides Wooop's bag. He made lots appreciative noises during the *cat scan*. Frank tells us, "Hey when I first saw you I thought, 'What the heck are they doing here?' Now I understand."

Week 3. As we enter we see that a student nurse is sitting with Audrey who is crying softly.

Audrey says, "So glad to see you, you will stop me making a fool of myself."

She obviously does not want to break down. I give her a *cat scan* and Heebie Jeebie massages the nurse. I give the nurse a soft brush so that she could stroke Audrey while Heebie Jeebie plays a calypso song, "Leave a little girl in Kingston Town." It is a rather sad song and her chins trembles. One tear runs down her cheek. Audrey says "Yes, but I do not want to cry." Then Heebie Jeebie suggests she make a request. She asks for a more cheerful song and names *"You are My Sunshine."* We all sing and Wooops whirls around the room with dreadful dancing with booted leg up through a huge rainbow silk banner. Audrey laughs, gives some dancing tips, and we all laugh again. Over the next few weeks we had many warm wonderful times. One rainy day we willingly had her photo taken with a ridiculously looking child's little yellow rain hat to match Wooops. It sat on her pinup board for the weeks to come.

Week 12. Audrey is now in a single room and unconscious–the fold out bed is a telltale sign that either Frank or Norma had stayed overnight with Audrey. They invite us in, accept shoulder massages and tell us about Audrey's life, how tough it had been, but also her love of jokes, her care of others and how she had loved our visits.

In Week 3, I had been tempted to leave her to have a cry with the nurse. We usually welcome tears but she voiced that, at this time, her need was to not cry. We had to trust that she knew what she wanted–music to uplifts her spirit. When Audrey was dying, Frank and Norma welcomed us and it was our privilege to be with them.

WE SEEK TO ELEVATE PEOPLE IN STATUS

We Seek to Express Solidarity with Humanity

We invite people to participate in many things that level us and connect us as humans. When we enter the nursing station, and staff ask for shoulder or head massages, it matters little who is a doctor or who is an orderly. We find that activities such as singing or playing coloured hand bells bring us together and emphasises our common humanity. When the moment calls for it, Dr. Heebie Jeebie hands out different coloured bells, each making a different note. He plays some himself and conducts so that people ring their bell at the right time. We have the usual "business of the clowns," which means the sillier one gets it wrong in some way, rearranging who has what coloured bells or playfully haggling over who is in charge, but we eventually get it right. Mistakes come naturally to the low status clown and it takes any pressure away from people to perform well. It seemed very satisfying to have a group do this together.

We Seek to Raise the Status of Those We Encounter by Lowering Our Own

These notes written about our time with Glad reflect this aspect of the work. She is beautiful dignified woman who has been slowly dying with great poise and we have sung songs over the past weeks. Recently, I, Wooops, had begun wearing pink baby trainers on her head and I notice that today Glad has a pink crocheted hat covering her hairless head, rendered bald from chemotherapy.

"Ooooh we should form the piiink hats society," croons Wooops as she enters the room. "Shall we let Heebie join; his red hat is sorta pink?"

Glad is quick to reply, "No he'll have to earn his way in."

She sounds and looks like a snotty schoolgirl with her raised nose and eyebrows. Heebie improvises a tune on his ukulele and sings with a bleating voice, "I have got a pink hat I reeeeeeeaally have." She makes many further requests and only later Glad softens her stance and says that she'll let Heebie Jeebie into our club if he can tell a joke. He obliges. She consents.

This week we learnt that she loves horses and so we talked about that. Then Wooops asked her the name of their current horse and this embarrasses her because she cannot recall it.

She replied rather sheepishly, "I hope that you forget words sometimes."

Wooops says proudly, "Well actually I am trying really, really hard to learn words to build up a big medical *constabulary* and I've even looking in the medical *Pictionary.*"

Glad smiled a wonderful smile. An onslaught of word mishaps brings laughter.

"I've really been trying hard you know, *constipating* on it."

We found our interaction fun because she chose to join in the game of the Pink Hats Society. We wanted to endow her with power to include or exclude. We found it very satisfying that instead of politeness she chose to exclude him and made him jump hoops to gain entry. Meanwhile, she had good reasons for us to sing and joke. We exposed a weakness in her, a faltering memory and so we needed to lower our own mental faculties in order to allow her to recovery her dignity. Clown comes from the word clod. So that even the most vulnerable might feel competent in the company of silly, clumsy clowns.

TO SENSITIVELY TAILOR HUMOUR, MUSIC, TOUCH, AND COLOUR TO THE INTERESTS OF THOSE WE ENCOUNTER

We Need to Respond to the Requests of Key Person

We do not engage everyone at Daw House. Often people are asleep, in pain, too ill, or do not understand what we are about. I share a time about when the person hesitated about seeing us.

Frank is in his sixties and new to Daw House. We poke our heads into his room. Wooops asks if we can we come in for a minute.

"Er . . . um. Yes but precisely one minute."

We enter and introduce ourselves. Wooops announces that our introductions have taken ten seconds and tells them that we can give Frank and his visitor each a massage for the remaining fifty seconds. Frank groans with pleasure at the massage and we begin to count down from ten. On the "blast off" we wave and leave.

Since we honoured his conditions of entry by carefully counting the seconds, Frank could relax. Later we learnt that he was waiting for pain relief. His initial negotiation invited us to play with the agreed sixty seconds. We were completely present with them for a rich, sparkling sixty seconds and were amazed how much fun and pleasure could happen in one minute. In dramatic jargon we accept "offers," make one of our own and then respond to the offer that follows. In other words we say, "yes" to whatever people offer us.

TO INVITE A SENSE OF WONDER AND SPONTANEITY

We met Anna from Russia. She seemed breathless and sleepy and since she did not lighten up, we decided to excuse ourselves saying that we would let her sleep. I announced, as I leapt clumsy ballet style out of her door, that here was a little Rudolph Nureyef for her. She laughed and stopped Heebie Jeebie from leaving by questioning him about the contents of each pocket. She then noticed his green ukulele. "Hey do you play the balinika?"

Heebie Jeebie improvised some Russian sounds and Wooops did the best imitation of Cossack dancing that she could muster. She seemed incredulous and wanted more. Heebie finished with "Fiddler on the Roof." She laughed and clapped.

"Ooh you play Russian music. . . . I know that one was the man on the roof."

The spontaneity and her joy made it very satisfying for us. We are full of wonder at the direction that our playful interactions take since they have an uncanny life of their own. Ideally, we follow whatever we are given.

TO TRANSFORM SITUATIONS
THROUGH THE IMAGINATION

A Blood Transfusion Becomes a Transformation to Royalty

Dr. Wooops noticed that Brian, who is very still and pale, has a bright red line giving him blood. I look him in the eye and say, "There is something wrong, it's most definitely the wrong colour. You need blue blood."

"Yes, yes, you're so right of course, the red blood helps me relate to commoners."

"Well it's obviously working, cos you are making us feel welcome," says Wooops.

After a few medical examinations of this royal person, we began to leave but since he was an important person we back our way out of room bowing and scraping.

"Is are you a Prince or a Lord or perhaps a Baron?"

Baron comes the answer.

We could hear him chuckling when we are two doors away. A week later he is out in a chair and the musician therapist plays the harp for him and it was so like a chamber scene from Henry the 8th that we bowed low with, "Court jester at your service My Lord." "Yes come, come, and sit here at my side,"

I put this in the category of one of our most spectacular interactions. What began as my attempt to cope with the sight of blood, became a wonderfully, dignifying interaction. We were surprised at his joy, and his willingness to enter imaginative play that elevated his status and briefly allowed him to transcend his suffering. Playfulness brings possibility of expressing solidarity with humanity, of spacious in our soul, wholeness of mind, body, spirit, and an affirmation of life in all its fullness.

To Allow Freedom of Expression of the Full Range of Emotions

Cathy, in her sixties, repeatedly told staff and volunteers exactly the same story of being discharged from a large public hospital without the promised help. The first time we met, she demanded that we turn off the overhead lights so we fumble about taking ages foolishly trying any button in the room. She does not acknowledge that we are clowns and wants to talk, although she playfully informs us that her name is "Dr. McGoolash." She says that she has a tough life and that her relationships with her children were strained. The next week begins with the same lament.

"Lets send, this deserves a tough letter," Says Wooops.

"Bah, needs more than a letter," she screws up her face in disdain at Wooops silly idea.

Wooops leans forward and says, "Yeah, but what if we sent a bomb in it?"

"I want a short jetty to line them all up and push them off," comes the reply, "I want the whole staff. . . . "

"Look you got just de righta person. . . . Let's get dem put cement in their boots. And them push them off that way they sink. They'll be sleeping with de fishes. . . . "

We see Cathy two weeks later. She gives us a knowing wink and remarks that it looks like we are in for some fun. We massage and in the midst of our conversation jetties come up. . . .

"Hey you supply the boots I'll supply the cement," says Wooops.

"Now you are talking," smiles Cathy.

Wooops put on Grouch Marx glasses to look tough. We plot.

"Yeah. Let's find the shortest dretty."

Cathy and TeapoT laugh heartily.

"Aw even when I'm trying to be tough, I get my words mixed up," complains Wooops.

More laughs and declare that it is time to celebrate the plan with some bubbly. I blow bubbles from the tiny champagne bottle. In a moment of dire inspiration turn the bubbles from champagne into air bubbles from the drowning victims.

"You know of course the further they go down the bigger the bubbles."

I bring out larger bubbles and then blow even larger ones from a champagne-size bottle of champagne bubbles . . . after a while they stop. We pause.

"Look they must have stopped breathing!!"

"Goood, goood.' She replies and falls asleep.

Cathy died two days later. It seems horrifying that innocent clowns engage in plots of mass murder. However, the thought of dire punishment seemed to satisfy her. It is obvious that Wooops makes an earnest but very pathetic Mafia. We are still clowns play-acting as tough guys. They laugh loudly when Wooops mixes her words because the world of clowning breaks out of the world of the Mafia. We all know that the whole plan is completely fanciful. Consequently, the grim schemes take full flight in the safe, dramatic, structured and controlled realm of play-acting that follows its own rules and temporarily suspends the harsh restraints of real life. The unique quality of imaginative play is that it eludes judgment. These games paradoxically combine sincerity and mirth, suspense and relaxation. The self-forgetting pleasure is in the game itself. The game is absorbing and yet at the same time the players transcend themselves and their games for it is after all only game.

DISCUSSION

Sometimes the intensity and direction of these interactions both delight and shock us. We ask ourselves "Are we going beyond the boundaries of play?" and "Why do they seem so satisfying and refreshingly powerful?" Sometimes it seems like pioneering work with adults because, while clown doctors are world wide, publications are sparse, and mostly about children. I (Thompson-Richards, 2003, pp. 206-208) did publish stories in the *European Journal of Palliative Care* in which Loraine, in the context of playing with plastic hammers as *anshethics*, asks us to knock her off. Wooops swallowed hard and then counted down from ten. On "Blastoff," Wooops announced that Loraine must be in heaven and all six flapped about pretending to be angels before collapsing in laughter. *She courageously addressed her death in front of her adult children.*

I was relieved and gratified to find confirmation for our work from Caroline Simmonds, a.k.a. Dr. Giraffe, from *Le Re Medicin*. Along with Bernie Warren, she chronicles the work of the French clowns with children who endure weeks of strict isolation and many traumatic procedures to receive bone marrow. Some relished getting one clown to doing dreadful things to the other. Caroline recognized their need to fancifully scapegoat others as catharsis for their experiences. The French clowns came across nurses desperately trying to bribe Rosa to take her pills. La Mouche offers to lock Dr. Giraffe in the dark closet if she, Rosa will take one pill. For the second pill she offers to pour ice water over Dr. Giraffe (2004, p. 53). Rosa takes one pill. From the closet Dr. Giraffe yells, "DO NOT TAKE THE PILL, DO NOT. . . . " Rosa takes the pill and Dr. Giraffe gets the ice water. The conductor-persecutor-victim games go on for months. Caroline Simmonds reminds us (Simmonds & Warren, 2004, p. 80) that the traditional role of the clown has been as scapegoat.

I also find reassurance from the Blatners (1988:29), leaders in their field of psychodrama and authors of *The Art of Play*, when they write

> The make believe play of childhood reflects the ability of the mind to create a special category experience called playfulness. The phenomenon of play, they say, involves a pleasurable paradox, a condition in which something is both real and not real at the same time. . . .

> Play allows the mind to operate at some distance from the task, because it used other category of "not really real" as a kind of laboratory for trying out different possibilities. . . . (1988, p. 125)

> They describe the process as "a mastery, aesthetic tension, cathartic, release, humorous amusement, and in short delight in discov-

ering the subtle cleverness of mentally manipulating perception and cognition. This pleasure is increased when it can be shared with others" (1988, pp. 30-31). They also write about the magic power of *if*, since it signals for the change of definition of reality-status.

How does this relate to spirituality? I trust that stories effuse with care of the spirit. I trust that the stories celebrate life and joy for their own sake; that they show that work and play are not separate categories; and that joy is not reserved for leisure but makes our whole existence shine. Jurgen Moltman (1975, p. 46) also says that "play goes beyond the categories of doing, having and achieving and leads us into the categories of being, of authentic human existence and demonstrative rejoicing in it." Berryman (1988, cover) writes "Many see playing as a superficial or trivial, act, but I see it as life giving act. It makes us young when we are old and matures us when we are young."

> Joy *is* the meaning of life. The most powerful image of joy for me is one of God playfully, exuberantly dancing with wild abandon in sheer delight over us (Zeph. 3:17). Moltman creatively substitutes the word *play* in Proverbs 8:30. *I am daily His delight, playing before Him always.* He asks about the purpose of humanity and answers from the Westminster Catechism of 1647 that the chief end of humanity is to glorify God and to enjoy Him forever. The point of life is joy. It brings the possibility of physical spontaneity, synthesis of our abilities, which in turn create in us a feeling of wellbeing. Joy brings about the possibility of expressing our common humanity; of creating spaciousness for our spirits; and shouts a definite "yes" to life in all its fullness. In the good times and bad the whole point of life is still joy.

CONCLUSION

So the work of Clown Doctors is to be purveyors of joy in the midst of suffering. The work is as rich and varied as the people we encounter. Finding joy means celebrating life and celebrating people–as people. It takes faith in humanity that behind what we see are people with the capacity for laughter and tears. Consolation comes when we truly connect with people so they may momentarily transcend their present circumstances. We do not always achieve our aims. As I concluded in the *Eu-*

ropean Journal of Palliative Care (2003 p. 208), "There are many wonderful, sparkling moments and times of profound connection with people that are interwoven with less spectacular but nevertheless warm, friendly times. At its best, caring clowning can speak the language of the heart, bring consolation, and touch the human spirit."

REFERENCES

Berryman, J. (1988). *Godly play: The way of religious education.* San Francisco: Harper.

Blatner, A., & Blatner, A. (1988). *The art of play: Helping adults reclaim imagination and spontaneity.* 1st ed. New York: Human Science Press.

Moltman, J. (1973). *Theology of joy.* London: SCM.

Simmonds, C., & Warren, B. (2004). *The clown doctor chronicles: At the interface/probing the boundaries.* Amsterdam: New York: Rodopi.

Thompson-Richards, J. (2003). Caring clowning as a healing art in palliative care. *European Journal of Palliative Care.* Sept/Oct, 10, 206-208.

Ageing and Death:
A Buddhist-Christian
Conceptual Framework
for Spirituality in Later Life

Ruwan Palapathwala, PhD

SUMMARY. With reference to the Buddhist idea of *anattā* (no-*self* or no-*soul*) and the Christian notion of *pneumā*, this essay outlines a conceptual framework for a meaningful spirituality in later life. It critically examines the importance of consumerist constructs of human life based on "life styles" which propagate a denial of ageing and death. The essay argues that the complementary visions of the nature of the self found in both Buddhism and Christianity suggests a Buddhist-Christian notion of *anattā-pneumā* which signifies the self-empty-spiritual life as a basis for spirituality in later life. *[Article copies available for a fee from The Haworth Document Delivery Service: 1-800-HAWORTH. E-mail address: <docdelivery@haworthpress.com> Website: <http://www.HaworthPress.com> © 2006 by The Haworth Press, Inc. All rights reserved.]*

Ruwan Palapathwala, PhD, is Lecturer, Pastoral Theology and Asian Religions, Trinity College Theological School, the University of Melbourne, United Faculty of Theology, the Melbourne College of Divinity.

Address correspondence to: Rev. Dr. Ruwan Palapathwala, Trinity College University of Melbourne, Royal Parade, Parkville Vic 3052, Australia (E-mail: ruwanp@trinity.unimelb.edu.au).

[Haworth co-indexing entry note]: "Ageing and Death: A Buddhist-Christian Conceptual Framework for Spirituality in Later Life." Palapathwala, Ruwan. Co-published simultaneously in *Journal of Religion, Spirituality & Aging* (The Haworth Pastoral Press, an imprint of The Haworth Press, Inc.) Vol. 18, No. 2/3, 2006, pp. 153-168; and: *Aging, Spirituality and Palliative Care* (ed: Elizabeth MacKinlay) The Haworth Pastoral Press, an imprint of The Haworth Press, Inc., 2006, pp. 153-168. Single or multiple copies of this article are available for a fee from The Haworth Document Delivery Service [1-800-HAWORTH, 9:00 a.m. - 5:00 p.m. (EST). E-mail address: docdelivery@haworthpress.com].

Available online at http://www.haworthpress.com/web/JRSA

doi:10.1300/J078v18n02_12

KEYWORDS. Ageing, suffering, death, spirituality, Buddhism, Christianity

In the context of our modern Western consumer-oriented culture it has become an arduous task to discuss ageing and death and spirituality in later life. This is particularly so because Christianity and its significant contribution to the Western civilisation's understanding of human life as a whole is both the substructure of our value systems and the impotent force that has fallen prey to consumerism. As a consequence, the basic templates of value systems that govern and order human life in general–and later life in particular–in our times reflect the ethos, ethics and goals of capital-base consumerism. It is for these reasons that the religio-cultural expectations of ageing and socioeconomic and political rhetoric concerning ageing are predominantly coloured with an emphasis on "lifestyle." With the increasing bureaucratisation of life the "quality" of caring for the ageing and dying has almost become synonymous with notions such as "client management" and "compliance with guidelines and standards."

The pathological obsessions with ageless youth and ideal body shapes which are propagated by the consumerist media have deprived people of graceful ageing and the acceptance of death. The human experience of suffering which is part of life is significantly reduced to a "condition" that could be "managed." These symptoms of our times have contributed to making old age and death significant enigmas for the ageing. In this environment, on the one hand, a meaningful spirituality for the ageing could be easily overlooked. On the other hand, it is also possible that spirituality could be offered to the ageing as another consumable product which could be "shopped for" in the vast market of spiritualities.

In this essay I seek to appraise the consumerist Christian approaches to understanding ageing, death, and spirituality and argue that a meaningful passage through ageing and death ultimately lies in a spirituality which is articulated in a view of life in its entirety, with reference to the Buddhist and Christian understanding of one's self in the Divine. This is achieved by demonstrating that the Buddhist and Christian notions of *anattā*[1] (no-soul or no-self) and *pneumā* (spirit) offer the basis for complementary visions of the nature of true self which enable us to understand human life and its stages–birth, youth, maturity, old age, and death–in perspective so that these stages may become the foundation for a meaningful spirituality in later life.

In spite of being the primary supplier of "cultural resources" to the modern Western consumer society, to a significant majority, Christianity has almost ceased to be a source of meaningful spirituality in later life. By cultural resources I mean the symbols, meanings, ideologies, and legitimacy that every cultural domain uses to justify its actions and directions which are necessary for its identity and existence. As an obvious example, it can be shown how Christianity provided "cultural resources" for the development of a capital-based market economy in the Western world.[2] Hence, in the same way as the narrative which gave the modern culture its legitimacy has crumbled, Christianity–which provided much of the "cultural resources" to that narrative–also has fragmented. Hence, its spiritual heritage, which continues to inform the substructure of the Western value system, cannot be revived without reference to–and without being in dialogue with–a religious tradition that did not go through the mill of modernity as Christianity did. This further justifies my choice of Buddhism–the Theravada tradition, in particular–as a point of reference.

SPIRITUALITY AND THE BUDDHIST-CHRISTIAN VIEW OF HUMAN LIFE

In a book on the cosmogonic myths of religious traditions (Palapathwala, 2005),[3] I have defined spirituality as our transcendental awareness about the "more" in us which seeks progression in and through our quest for our "where from" and "where to." Our quest for the "where from," I have argued, is the most fundamental wonderment and angst we have in us for having been born in this world and knowing that old age and death are its natural end. Our quest for the "where to" is the fundamental search for answers to that experience so that we may overcome from that state of angst and fear of being.

That awareness is transcendental because the spiritual quest–although an important aspect of our bodily existence–is not ultimately limited to, or defined by, life's vicissitudes, greatness and tragedy. This awareness, I have argued, comes from the *More* in us which is the dimension of true *self–anattā* or *pneumā*–the Seat of the Divine. That dimension is what I call *spiritual*. Our search for it–the *quest*–is the experience which forms the basis for what is known as *spirituality*. I have demonstrated that, since this dimension lies at the depth of all the spheres of a culture, the life of a human being, consciously or sub-consciously, is lived with reference to this dialectical tension between our quest for "where from" and our quest for "where to." If the spiritual meaning of life could be viewed this way, it is only through a progressive quest after our *"where from"* and *"where to"* that life may receive its meaning with an increasing recognition of the *More* in us.

Maggam bhāveti, "making the way to become," is the phrase found in Buddhist scriptures that describe this life process. According to Buddhism, this process is a spiritual quest which entails one's increasing understanding of the true nature of the phenomenal world and life (*bhavā*) so that one may attain *nibbana* (or *nirvāna* in Sanskrit; *ni* negation and *vāna* craving). In the Christian Bible, St. Paul alludes to the same process when he refers to the necessity that we all should *"reach unity in the faith and in the knowledge of the Son of God and become mature, attaining to the whole measure of the fullness of Christ"* (Ephesians 4:13).

If the scriptures of Buddhism and Christianity highlight the significance of a progressive *becoming*, it could be argued that human life becomes meaningful only if the successive stages in life–infancy, childhood, adulthood, old age, and death–are advanced with an increasing knowledge and recognition of the true nature of *self*, the source from which spirituality springs. The recognition of the true nature of *self* entails a depth of understanding which accepts the conditions to which the physical body is subjected to: ageing, suffering and death.

When the issue is looked at in this way, it seems unnecessary to discuss how Buddhism and Christianity view ageing and death for the reason that the general themes which are associated with ageing and death in both religious traditions–illness, suffering, and *dis*-ease, for instance–are only accessory to explaining the phenomenon of the human condition and its purpose and aim: deliverance from sin (Christianity) and a deluded understanding of existence (Buddhism). In the *Abhidhamma Pitaka* (the Higher Teaching of Buddha), for example, one will not find references to persons or objects as I, we, he, she, man, woman, tree, lake, etc. Such persons and objects, the exposition in the *Abhidhamma Pitaka* considers are relative concepts. Thus, only their ultimate elements are analysed and precisely defined in terms of *khandhas*–the five instruments of clinging to existence–to describe the transient psycho-physical phenomena which are subject to change, are tainted with suffering and without substance.

It is only in the general teaching of the nature of these psycho-physical phenomena in the *Suttanta Pitaka* is it demonstrated how human beings who are made up of the five instruments of clinging are ignorant of the true nature of existence, subjecting themselves to birth (*jāti*), decay and old age (*jarā*), disease (*vyādhi*) and death (*marana*). Thus, the fundamental purpose of Buddha's teaching was to enlighten human beings about the true nature of all *dukkha*-laden phenomena which is without permanence and substance–a permanent ego-centred self–so that they may seek deliverance. The Pali word, *du-kkha* means difficult to endue, incapable of satisfying: always changing, incapable of truly fulfilling us or making us happy. It also means unease, anxiety, collective-anxiety, physical, and emotional pain, and 'ill' in the sense of its use in Old English. Enlightenment about this condition alone can give knowledge about all phenomena and enable us to understand old age and death in perspective and thereby attain *nibbāna*, the deathless, which is possible only through wayfarering towards the highest *self* which is the ego-less self.

In the Christian understanding, *"the wages of sin is death"* (Romans 6:23) and hence death is the final outcome of living in a sinful world. Therefore, according to St. Paul, "The last enemy to be destroyed is death," and *"when Christ returns death will be swallowed up in victory"* (1 Corinthians 15:26, 54-55). This ultimate experience of death for a Christian is seen in related ways: suffering, ageing, illnesses, and other such calamities. However, besides implicitly representing Jewish views that suffering is due to punishment or retribution to sin, the New Testament, on which the Christian teaching is predominantly based, does not give an explanation why suffering exists in the world. Christianity affirms that suffering is intrinsic to all phenomena of the world: *"For we know that the whole creation groans and labours with birth pangs together until now"* (Romans 8:22).

The Gospels assert that Jesus faced suffering but was not defeated by it at any rate. While the temptations of Jesus and his Passion are clear indications of his encounter with suffering, his healing of people with physical and spiritual ailments and his own resurrection vindicate his victory over suffering. According to the teachings of the New Testament, as exemplified in the life of Jesus, an intimate relationship with God enables the Christian to endure suffering without losing God in the experience. Through that experience Christians respond to suffering with *agape* (unconditional love).

Death completes our changing process, and the whole experience of ageing and death is a part of God's work within us. Then, the most primary concern is our victory over death when *"God shall wipe away all tears from our eyes; and there shall be no more death, neither sorrow, nor crying, neither shall there be any more pain"* (Revelations 21:4). This becomes possible only by our being faithful to God unto death so that God can give us the crown of life (Revelations 2:10) which He can do only if we have come to live a self-emptying spiritual life in God through Christ.

THE WEST AND THE SELF

The difficulty we are faced with in the contemporary West, however, is to understand this "true self" as a basis for spirituality not only in later life but also in early life. This is due to our present experience of the world which has come to obscure the relevance of any understanding of *self*.

For instance, in the main, there are five important themes that critics of contemporary culture employ to demonstrate this loss of *self*. They argue that:

1. The idea of a *self* achieved under modernity has disappeared in the wake of consumerism, mass culture, and the growing bureaucratisation of life. What matters ultimately is not any transcendental reality which fashions one's life, but images. The "authentic *self*" does not matter any longer; what authenticates one's self are fashion statements, shopping, and lifestyles (e.g., Jameson, 1999; Baudrillard, 1998; and Debord, 1990).

2. The idea of *self* in contemporary society is related to the question of identity and how the increasing invasion of signs and images in the media, displays, advertising, and so on have created ideal lifestyles or sub cultural narratives about which people may fantasise and with which they can identify. As a direct consequence of this, *self* and identity have become something for which one "shops" (e.g., Kellner, 1989; McRobbie, 1991, 1994).

3. The claim for a stable, unified *self* has always been an illusion. The modern-day notion of the self is bound up with, and inseparable from, complex operations of power in a given society (e.g., Foucault, 1980; Janicki, 1999).

4. Essential definitions of *self* are tied up only with gender (him/her, he/she, etc.), and language could be used in experimental ways to encourage multiple forms of selfhood (Kristeva, 1989, 1991).

5. The phenomena of artificial intelligence, computer simulations, and the hybrids of humans and machines have further removed the relevance of an authentic *self*.[4]

These profound changes in society have altered the way in which our society has come to view ageing, old age, and death. The images and subcultural narratives continually feed in beliefs which are contrary to the true nature of all things. It is in this context that a Buddhist-Christian understanding of the nature of true *self* could become the basis of a meaningful spirituality in later life.

SEMANTIC DIFFICULTIES WITH SELF, SOUL, SPIRIT, AND ANATTĀ

Before the relevance of the notion of *self* in Buddhist and Christian canonical literature could be examined as a conceptual basis for spirituality, these terms need semantic clarification for three reasons:

  i. the limitations of the English translations of the Pali and Greek words *attā* and *pneumā*;
 ii. the two terms are used interchangeably with corresponding terms such as "mind," "soul," and "individual" in both Buddhist and Christian canonical as well as non-canonical literature; and
iii. the attempt to outline the semantics of the words themselves will illustrate the poststructuralist claim for the instability of words, concepts, and meanings.

From even a cursory reading of literature that may be termed "Western," irrespective of whether on the arts or the sciences, one cannot but notice the repeated use of terms such as *soul, self, spirit,* and *mind*. However, in each piece of writing the connotations and nuances that the words carry differ. For instance, the notion of *soul* in the writings of Aristotle is used simply to refer to the form of the body. However, for Plato, most Christian theologians of the first millennium CE, Descartes and many others, *soul* is the immaterial "part" of the body which is temporarily united with the material body (Honderich, 1995, p. 841). Then the word *mind*–which is sometimes used interchangeably with *soul*–is used in two senses. In the first sense *mind* is taken to refer to the *self* or subject that thinks, feels, and so on, and is thus related to an organism.

In the second sense, *mind* is used as a generic term to refer to the metaphysical substance which pervades all individual minds (Woods, 1982, p. 214). The term *self*, although normally used interchangeably with "person," lays more emphasis on the "inner," or the psychological dimension of personality than on its outward bodily form. Hence a *self* is conceived to be the subject of consciousness. In Western philosophy, a distinction is drawn between substantive and non-substantive theories of *self*. While the former refer to *self* as a substance–physical or non-physical–the latter is considered in terms of a mode of substance. Hence for Hume, *self* is nothing but a bundle of different perceptions, and *self*, for him, belongs to the category of modes (Parft, 1984).

The Greek word *pneumā*, which is translated as spirit, literally means *breath*. However, sometimes Greeks used the term to refer to air, as well as to the breath of the cosmos. Aristotle believed that heat in *pneumā* caused the sensitive soul to be transmitted to an embryo located near the heart in the mature organism, serving to mediate movement and perception. For the Stoics, spirit is a fine, subtle body forming the soul of the cosmos. It also helps in explaining growth, behavior, and rationality.

The senses of the term *pneumā* that are useful for this essay are those found in the New Testament. W.D. Stacey has distinguished six senses of *pneumā* in the Pauline literature: *Pneumā*

- i. as applied to the Divine–to God, to the Holy Spirit, and to the Spirit of Christ;
- ii. as a divine influence in the lives of believers, creating in them "spiritual gifts";
- iii. as applied to "seducing spirits" in opposition to the Divine Spirit;
- iv. as the evil influence which issued from the disobedient spirits;
- v. as a purely Christian spirit created in the believer which enables him/her to commune with God because spirit can meet with spirit;
- vi. as "the natural possession of every man, which of itself, is neither good nor bad, and is not easily distinguished from *psychē*" (Stacey, 1956, pp. 128-129).

The senses of *pneumā* numbered (i) and (v) are of immediate relevance to the argument presented in this essay.

The Buddhist word *attā* in Pali and the corresponding word *ātman* in Sanskrit basically mean *self*. There are also other terms in the Vedic sources in Sanskrit for *self* such as *jīva* (life), *jīvatman* (life-breath), *purusha* (the essence that is deposited in the body), and *ksetrajna* (one who knows the body). When the negative prefix "*an*" is added, the term *attā* qualifies itself to mean non-*atta* or no-*self*. As in the case of the words *soul*, *spirit*, and *psychē* in Western literature, in the early Vedic hymns, the Sanskrit word *ātman* too had assumed the connotation of "breath." This "breath" was thought of as some "life force" that could leave–and return to–the body. It has been argued that in this connection the word for mind–*manas*–which can be translated as *self* and also as *consciousness* can be seen as a synonym for *ātman* and that association gradually developed and gave rise to the concepts of *self* which we find in the Upanishads. The central concept of Vedantic thought for Ultimate Reality is *Brahman*, which is *Brahma*–when personified–and is known as the Great Self or Great Soul. In the Vedic literature every human being has a "little self " or a "little *ātman*" which is the same as *Brahman's* which may come to union with the Ultimate through self-realisation (Radhakrishnan, 1999, pp. 151-172). It seems that this is the immediate context from which the many theories concerning this *ātman* came to be developed before the time of Buddha (*c*. 600 BCE). Possibly it is these developments that contributed to the fact that the Pali word *attā* also has the nuances of self, soul, body, person, and mind.

The Pali Buddhist philosophical term for *individual* is *santāna*, that is, a flux or continuity (of the *khandhas*–the five instruments of clinging). It includes the mental and physical elements as well. The *kammic* force of each individual binds the elements together. This uninterrupted flux or continuity of the psychophysical phenomenon (*nāma-rupā*), which is conditioned by *kamma*, and not limited only to the present life, having its source in the beginningless past and its continuation into the future–had been wrongly understood as the Buddhist substitute for the *permanent ego* or the *immortal soul*, especially in Christian literature (Jayatilleke, 1975). Of these various Pali words the term *attā* for *self* and *anattā* for no-*self* are relevant to this essay.

BUDDHISM AND THE SELF

The way in which the Buddhist notion of *anattā* helps us in the context of speaking about the human person and spirituality is through its critique of every false construct of *self*. In the Buddhist Canon the notion of no-*self* is related to the ideas of impermanence (*aniccā*) and suffering (*dukkha*), and together they represent the Buddhist description of the state of affairs which poses the question, as I have called it: "where from?"

A simplified representation of the interrelatedness of these three concepts can be described thus: because of the impermanent nature of all that is, craving and attachment–which give rise to the deluded understanding that *self* is permanent or has substance–form the precondition for the *dukkha*-laden psychophysical phenomenon, the human phenomenon, which is composed of the five groups (*upādānakhandha*) that facilitate our clinging to the phenomenal world:

i. mind and matter (*nāma-rūpa*);
ii. sensations *(vedanā)*;
iii. perceptions (*saññā*);
iv. mental formations (*samkhāra*); and
v. consciousness (*viññāna*).

Thus, in Buddha's famous second sermon (which is called the *anattālakkhana sutta*, Oldenburg, 1879) the idea of *anattā* is clearly explained by dismissing step by step the view that each group of clinging cannot be *self*; for example, the body (or matter) cannot be the *self*, for if it were, then the body would not be subject to disease and one would be able to control one's body at pleasure, the *self* being assumed as autonomous. The same argument is applied to the other four groups of clinging: the sensations, perceptions, mental formations (or dispositions), and consciousness. The sermon concludes with Buddha's showing that when one realises that all these groups of clinging are not the *self*, one would turn away from them and by eradication of all desire one would attain release.

Release is the attainment of *nibbāna*, the "where to." Nibbana is the state in which the turmoil of the groups of clinging that is brought about through birth, old age, disease, and death–the causes of suffering–ceases. In other words, when the causes of mundane wanderings–the five groups of clinging–are destroyed, what remains is nothing other than the pure Self. The pure Self, in effect, is *nibbāna*. *Nibbāna* is not annihilation. In the older texts of the Buddhist *Pali* Canon, *nibbāna* is compared to "fire going out," rather than to "fire being put out" (De Silva, 1975, p. 68). The obvious point of the sermon is that the five groups of clinging are not *self* and that the knowledge and the pursuit of real *self* alone provide the framework within which to view human existence in its entirety and its purpose in perspective. When the concept of *anattā* is seen in this way it could be stated that the spirituality Buddhism cultivates is based on the search for the true *self*.

There are many other instances in the Pali Canon that uphold this position in different ways. The teaching about the false view of the *self* appears in a tedious scholastic form in *Nikāyās* such as *Majjhima Nikāyā*[5] and *Samyutta Nikāyā* where, by employing permutations and combinations, twenty theories concerning the possible identification of the *self* with one, or more, or all of the five groups of clinging are disclosed and refuted. The dialogue between Sariputta and Yamaka in the *Samyutta Nikāyā* is an example.[6] It is also of interest to note that there is no mention of the doctrine of *self* in the *Brahmajala Sutta*[7] which outlines the heresies.

If this is the case, why is it that the later developments in Buddhism came to negate the *self* in a final way? While "orthodox Theravada Buddhist" scholars such as Walpola Rahula hold views to the contrary (Rahula, 1959), Rhys Davids (1978), a well-known authority on Buddhism, argues that the search for the *self* inwardly, which is one in nature with the Highest–the *"progressive revelation of a More in man"* in the Upanishads, the pursuit seen as the Way leading to *Brahman*, the Ultimate, was the teaching that Buddha taught and on which he expanded (Davids, 1978).[8] Davids also refers to that *"More in man"* as "God-in-Man," "Divine Selfhood," "Very God," and *Mahattam* (the Great Self) (Davids, 1978, pp. 12,13, 55). Agreeing on the fact that the *self* cannot be found in the five groups of clinging, she highlights two aspects of the early teaching which, she says, were Buddha's original contribution to the existing teaching of the Upanishads: (i) that "the true Becoming (where comes no decay) is in every man, the spirit the soul"; and (ii) substituting the Upanishadic teaching of attaining the splendid human knowledge of "I am, Thou art" (Sanskrit: *"Tat tvam asi"*) from a static state of "being That" to the dynamic.

"For the rapt complacency Buddha taught the divine unrest of the inner urge we call "duty," "conscience," and which India, though not then in religious terms, called *Dharma* (that which should be "borne," in mind, in heedfulness)" (Davids, 1978, p. 21) The outcome of this transition from the static to the dynamic is, she claims, that *Dharma*[9] in Buddhism came to take prominence over the idea of *self* in the Brahmanic teaching.

THE BIBLE, CHRISTIANITY, AND THE SELF

When the Bible is looked at from this perspective, it is clear that the Biblical and Buddhist notions of *self* not only correspond very closely, but that indeed, they are identical. In fact, there is the possibility of speaking of a Christian doctrine of *anattā* (De Silva, 1975, pp. 72-74).

The Biblical teaching of the creation of human beings by God highlights two truths: that the human being was made in God's image; and since the human being is a created being, the creature has the intrinsic character of not-being, if not absolute impermanence (*aniccā*). Human beings' creatureliness corroborates the truth expressed by the Buddhist doctrine of *anattā*.

The Old Testament Hebrew term *nephesh* corresponds to the New Testament notion of *psychē* (Greek) which, in the main, refers to the "life force" of living creatures. With reference to the Greek term for the carnal body–*sarx*–and the notion of *psychē* (and also *nephesh*), it is possible to demonstrate the psychophysical unity of the human being, apart from God's Spirit, as *psychē-sarx*, which bears a close resemblance to the Buddhist *nāma-rūpa* analysis of the human being (DeSilva, 1975, p. 80).

> Just as in Buddhism the human being is a unity of *nāma-rūpa*, so in the Bible the human being is a unity of *psychē-sarx*; just as Buddhism says that there is no soul entity within the *nāma-rūpa* complex, so the Bible leaves no room for a notion of an immortal soul within the *psychē-sarx* unity of the human being. Thus we could, in a sense, speak of a biblical doctrine of *anattā*. We could put the matter thus: Psychosomatic creatureliness is *anattā* (i.e., soulless and substanceless). . . . [In this way] not only would Christianity deny an ego entity but also exclusive individuality, so that it could be said that the person (*puggala*) thought of in purely individualistic terms in his singularity and independence does not in reality exist and cannot exist. If such a state were possible it could be described by the metaphors, *dust, shadow,* and *mist.* (De Silva, 1975, pp. 80-81)

What is apparent here is that the human being as *psychē-sarx* is substanceless and distinguished only from not being lifeless (*apsychē*). Then, while *psychē* is the life the human being shares with animals, the life that the human being alone can live is *pneumā*. This contrast is expressed in 1 Corinthians 15:45: "the first Adam became a living being (*psychē*), the last Adam became a life-giving spirit (*pneumā*). *Psychē* then denotes the life separated from God while *pneumā* expresses life derived from God. According to St. Paul, this separated *self* is the "carnal self "; and as far as the *self* is genuinely related to God it is spiritually minded and becomes *true self* (Romans 8:5-8) (De Silva, p. 84).

Humanity is not made immortal but is made for immortality, which is *not* a natural possession of the human being. God alone is eternal and it is only in relation to the eternal that we can be eternal. We are a unity of creatureliness and God-likeness; in other words, a unity of *anattā* and *pneumā*. *Anattā* indicates our organic nature; the fact that within the psycho-physical organism there is no permanent immortal entity and that as such, we are subject to old age, suffering, and death which are the marks of *dukkha* and *anicca*.

Pneumā indicates that extra dimension of being which makes us more than just a physical organism or a psycho-somatic complex. *Pneumā* is not another substance or a thing; it is rather the dynamic quality which makes the human being a person in his or her total experience of life: birth, ageing, suffering, and death. *Anattā-pneumā* signifies the self-empty-spiritual life (De Silva, p. 84), where there is no decay.

It is in these ways, then, that the notion of *pneumā* could be seen as Divine Spirit–which is the key to our understanding of the human being's spirit–"a purely Christian spirit created in the believer which enables him/her to hold communion with God because spirit with spirit can meet." This is the "transcendental dimension" of *pneumā* which, like *anattā*, can realise *nibbāna*–the "state" in which no-*self* is completely transcended and the *self* is realised, that is the "losing oneself in communion with Reality [God]"(De Silva, p. 84).

A BUDDHIST-CHRISTIAN FRAMEWORK FOR SPIRITUALITY

As the foregoing discussion has demonstrated, the Buddhist and Christian concepts of *anattā* and *pneumā* serve as imperatives to understand the conditions of human existence–ageing, suffering, and death–and the place of spirituality in life generally and in later life specifically. When examined, the meanings of *anattā* and *pneumā* with reference to the question of "where from" which signifies the quest for *self*–the *More* in us–as the ultimate aim in life, the "where to," have provided a broader framework to articulate a spirituality that informs a holistic view of life and its natural progress from birth to death.

This framework for spirituality in later life underlines three significant areas for consideration in the caring for people in later life. Firstly, the pastoral care of the ageing needs to take a much broader perspective of human life and its aim. This is important as the peoples of the world continue to be drawn further and further into one vast materialistic and consumer-oriented society; our experience of life continues to be limited to narrow segments of institutionalised existence. These fleeting and segmented experiences of life either disturb or completely eradicate one's view of life in its entirety and the understanding of the natural process of ageing and the cessation of physical existence in death.

Secondly, to keep the understanding of the human condition in perspective; in particular it means keeping the experience and the understanding of suffering as an ingredient of human existence. God is not to be blamed for suffering, for suffering is not punishment or retribution for sin. Buddhist and Christian understanding of human life demonstrates that ageing, suffering, and death are real and are universal and intrinsic to all conditioned phenomena. Knowing this gives life transformative power. Herein lies the quest for the "More"–the potentiality of humanity. It entails accepting, not resisting or denying, the natural processes of ageing, suffering, and death. To resist or deny is to succumb to the forces of consumerism.

Lastly, to recognise that the spirituality which is imperative in later life is not a consumer specific "product." It is a spirituality that needs to be understood, cultivated, and harnessed in later life in the light of one's total experience of life with a special emphasis on empowering one to accept and participate in the human experience of ageing. In actual fact, the spirituality which should instruct one in later life is the same spirituality that sustained one's youth; it only has matured with understanding of the human condition into new horizons. The ability on the part of the carer to enable the ageing person to be nurtured in a meaningful spirituality and the person receiving the caring to accept life in its stages of decline is to be empowered–that is, *the way to become* made possible–to anchor oneself to one's *anattā-pneumā*, the Seat of God and the wellspring of *nibbāna*, the deathless.

NOTES

1. The Buddhist words used in this essay are in *Pali.*

2. Historians such as Max Weber and–lately–Randall Collins, have shown the extent of the church's role in the birth and the flowering of capitalism. While Max Weber located the origin of capitalism in Protestant cities following the European Enlightenment, Randall Collins has shown that capitalism had already existed in the Middle Ages in rural areas, where monasteries–especially those of the Cistercians (Religious of the Order of Cîteaux, a Benedictine reform, established at Cîteaux in 1098 by St. Robert, Abbot of Molesme in the Diocese of Langres)–began to rationalise economic life.

According to Collins, it was the church that established what Max Weber called the "preconditions of capitalism." These include the rule of law and a bureaucracy for resolving disputes rationally, a specialised and mobile labour force, the permanence of institutions which enabled transgenerational investment and sustained intellectual and physical efforts, together with the accumulation of long-term capital, and a zest for discovery, enterprise, wealth creation, and new undertakings. By the time of the Enlightenment in the eighteenth century the capitalist ethos was so well established that it was able to flourish in a more secular environment with religion facing diminution in the post-Enlightenment years to follow. Collins, R. (1985). *Max Weber: A skeleton key.* California: Sage Publications, Inc.

3. Palapathwala, R. (2005). *Myths of origin and end: Pathways to interfaith dialogue.* Melbourne: CSIRID and Kerala, India: The Cosmic Community Centre and Dr. Alexander Mar Thoma Centre for Dialogue Kottarakara.

4. Marge Piercy (1991) presents an alarming scenario in her fascinating novel: *He, She or It.* Knopf: New York. In describing human beings with extensive computerised parts, she implies the possibility of obscuring the boundary between human beings and robots with software which has been engineered to understand humans,

5. Pali Text Society, (Ed.). (1888-1902), *Majjhima nikāyā,* ch. I, 138, 300 and *Samyutta nikaya.* (1884-1904), ch. iii. 66; iv. 34.

6. Pali Text Society (Ed). *Samyutta nikāyā.* (1884-1904), ch. ii. 13; 62.

7. Pali Text Society (Ed). (1890-1911), *Digha nikāyā,* ch. i. 1ff.

8. Davids, R. (1978). *Outlines of Buddhism.* New Delhi: Oriental Books Reprint Corporation, pp. 8-9, 19-20. Rhys Davids was the wife of the eminent Buddhist scholar Prof. T.W. Rhys Davids.

9. *Dhamma* in Pali.

REFERENCES

Baudrillard, J. (1998). *The consumer society: Myths and structures.* London: SAGE Publications.

Davids, R. (1978). *Outlines of Buddhism.* New Delhi: Oriental Books Reprint Corporation, 8-9, 19-20.

Debord, G. (1990). *Comments on the society of the spectacle.* London; New York: Verso.

De Silva, L. A. (1975). *The problem of the self in Buddhism and Christianity.* Colombo: The Centre for the Study of Religion and Society.

Foucault, M. (1980). *Power/knowledge*. Brighton, Sussex: Harvester Press.

Honderich, T. (Ed.). (1995). *Oxford companion to philosophy*. Oxford: Oxford University Press, p. 841.

Jameson, F. (1999). Postmodernism, or, the cultural logic of late capitalism. Durham: Duke University Press, (1998). *The cultural turn: Selected writings on the postmodern*, 1983-1998. London; New York: Verso.

Janicki, K. (1999). *Against essentialism*. Munchen: Loncom Europa.

Jayatilleke, K. (1975). *The message of Buddha*. London: George Allen & Unwin Ltd.

Kellner, D. (1989). *Critical theory, Marxism and modernity*. Cambridge: Polity.

Kristeva, J. (1991). *Strangers to ourselves*. New York and London: Harvester Wheatsheaf.

Kristeva, J. (1989). *Language–The unknown*. New York: Columbia University Press.

McRobbie, A. (1994). *Postmodernism and popular culture*. London, New York: Routledge.

McRobbie, A. (1991). *Feminism and youth culture: From 'Jackie' to 'just seventeen.'* Houndmills, Basingstok, Hampshire: Macmillan.

Oldenberg (Ed.). (1879). *Mahavagga. vinaya pitaka 1*. London, ch. i.6. 38ff.

Palapathwala, R. (2005). *Myths of origin and end: Pathways to interfaith dialogue*. Melbourne: CSIRID and Kerala, India: The Cosmic Community Centre and Dr. Alexander Mar Thoma Centre for Dialogue Kottarakara.

Pali Text Society Dictionary, p. 363, cited by De Silva, L. (1975), p. 68.

Pali Text Society (Ed). (1890-1911), *Digha nikāyā*, ch. i. 1ff.

Pali Text Society (Ed). *Samyutta nikāyā* (1884-1904), ch. ii. 13; 62.

Pali Text Society (Ed.). (1888-1902), *Majjhima nikāyā*, ch. I, 138, 300 and *Samyutta nikaya* (1884-1904), ch. iii. 66; iv. 34.

Parft, D. (1984) *Reasons and persons*. London: Oxford University Press.

Piercy, M. (1991). *He, she, and it*. New York: Knopf.

Radhakrishnan, S. (1999). *Indian philosophy* volume 1. New Delhi: Oxford University Press, pp.151-172.

Rahula, W. (1959). *What Buddha taught*. London: Gordan Frazer.

Stacey, W. (1956). The pauline view of man in relation to its Judaic and Hellenistic background. London: Macmillan & Co., Ltd., pp.128-129, cited in De Silva, L. (1975). *The problem of the self in Buddhism and Christianity*. Colombo: The Centre for the Study of Religion and Society, p. 83.

Janicki, K. (1999). *Against essentialism*. Munchen: Loncom Europa.

Williams, B. (1973). *Problems of the self*. Cambridge: Cambridge University Press.

Wood, L. (1982). *Dictionary of philosophy*. New York: Philosophical Library Inc., p. 214.

The 'Connection' Health Care Providers Make with Dying Patients

Ann Harrington, RN, DNE, BEd, MNg, PhD, FCN, FRCNA

SUMMARY. The literature confirms illness and hospitalisation can become spiritual encounters for patients and their families. Further, it has been established that both patients and their families are better equipped to deal with loss and change if they have a healthily developed spiritual sense of self. The aim of the study sought to determine the benefit or otherwise of a previous model of spiritual care. It asked 'from the perspective of the nurse and other health care providers, what constitutes spiritual care giving?' An ethnography was undertaken where data consisted of field notes, interviews, records, and diary entries. This paper reports on interview data, from which themes were derived. The major theme titled *their space* is expressed via a new model of spiritual care. It was shown that when caring for patients and their relatives, nurses and other health care professionals enter the world of the other to determine the other's needs. In so doing they typify agapé (altruistic love), where the individual cares for a complete stranger as if that stranger were family. This *connection* with the patient and their family is the foundation for spiritual care. *[Article copies available for a fee from The Haworth Document Delivery Service: 1-800-HAWORTH. E-mail address: <docdelivery@haworthpress.com> Website: <http://www.HaworthPress.com> © 2006 by The Haworth Press, Inc. All rights reserved.]*

Ann Harrington, RN, DNE, BEd, MNg, PhD, FCN, FRCNA, is Senior Lecturer, School of Nursing & Midwifery, Flinders University, Adelaide, SA, Australia.

[Haworth co-indexing entry note]: "The 'Connection' Health Care Providers Make with Dying Patients." Harrington, Ann. Co-published simultaneously in *Journal of Religion, Spirituality & Aging* (The Haworth Pastoral Press, an imprint of The Haworth Press, Inc.) Vol. 18, No. 2/3, 2006, pp. 169-185; and: *Aging, Spirituality and Palliative Care* (ed: Elizabeth MacKinlay) The Haworth Pastoral Press, an imprint of The Haworth Press, Inc., 2006, pp. 169-185. Single or multiple copies of this article are available for a fee from The Haworth Document Delivery Service [1-800-HAWORTH, 9:00 a.m. - 5:00 p.m. (EST). E-mail address: docdelivery@ haworthpress.com].

doi:10.1300/J078v18n02_13

KEYWORDS. Spiritual, spirituality, hospice, dying, ethnography, agape

INTRODUCTION, LITERATURE REVIEW
AND BACKGROUND TO THE STUDY

The literature confirms illness and hospitalisation can become spiritual encounters for patients and their families (Bolmsjo, 2000; Ross, 1994). Bown and Williams (1993) claim 'illness, suffering, and death . . . challenge personal meaning systems and intensify the search to make sense of life' (1993, p. 50). Further, it has been found that both patients and families (however defined) are better equipped to deal with loss and change if they have a healthily developed spiritual sense of self (Harrington, 2003).

Within Western literature certain authors argue that the terms 'spiritual' and 'spirituality' have lost their meaning since removal from their theistic roots (Bradshaw, 1997; Grenz, 1996; Brittain, 1986; Ellis, 1980). Such roots include the practice of a particular religion and the acknowledgment of a God dimension. Latterly however, Western literature confirms agreement among authors that spirituality is *not only* religious practice but that religious practice *may* be included as an expression of spirituality (Smith & McSherry, 2004; Draper & McSherry, 2002; Baldacchino & Draper, 2001; Hamilton, 1998; Froggatt, 1997; Oldnall, 1996; Harrington, 1995; Emblem & Halstead, 1993; Harrison, 1993; Mickley, Soeken, & Belcher, 1992; Fahlberg & Fahlberg, 1991). It should be noted some Eastern countries would not draw this distinction.

Most recently, spirituality has been expressed as a search for *meaning,* linking spirituality to the provision of meaning in/of life. Authors who agree that *spirit, spiritual, spirituality,* or the *spiritual dimension* encompass a search for meaning are many (Baldacchino & Draper, 2001; McSherry, 2000; Byrne, 1999; Fryback & Reinert, 1999; Narayanasamy, 1999; McSherry & Draper, 1998; Dyson, Cobb, & Forman, 1997; Relf 1997; Fry & Tan, 1996; Groer, O'Connor & Droppleman, 1996; Johnson-Taylor, Highfield, & Amenta, 1994; Harrison, 1993; Emblen, 1992). Groer, O'Connor, and Droppleman (1996), without elaborating on the time frame of their search, write of their review of 250 articles that found 75% equated spirituality with 'a personal philosophy of meaning' (1996, p. 376).

This intangibility of spirituality provided one of the triggers for a previous study (within a Masters degree) seeking registered nurses' perceptions of spiritual care (Harrington, 1993).

At that time four research questions were posed. These were:

1. What is meant by spiritual care?
2. What is undertaken as spiritual care?
3. What is the status of spiritual care in relation to normal care?
4. How adequate is education to its implementation?

The outcome of that study led to the generation of a *Spiritual Care Model* (Figure 1) which offered some guidance into practices deemed 'spiritual' (Harrington, 1995).

The respondents within this earlier study were all nurses. Therefore, the model gave recognition to the pivotal role played by the nurse (hence the unbroken line). Patients, seeking spiritual answers to questions, acknowledge the constant presence of the nurse. It is the nurse who is available to the patient 24 hours a day and there is acceptance that nurses act as 'brokers' to chaplaincy services. Bolmsjo (2000) found that patients request that nurses discuss spiritual issues and Cressey and Winbolt-Lewis (2000) argue that spiritual care is neither the

FIGURE 1. *Spiritual Care Model*

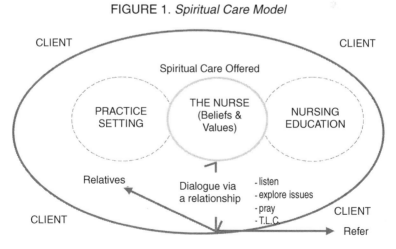

Spiritual Care Model. From Harrington, A. (1995) 'Spiritual Care: What Does it Mean to RNs?' AJAN 12, 4, pp. 5-14. Reprinted with permission.

sole responsibility and province of chaplains working within a religious framework nor 'only connected with death and dying' (2000, p. 170).

However, the other two features of this earlier model, the 'environment' within which practice occurs and 'educational preparation,' impact on the nurse's ability to offer spiritual care. That is, a supportive environment and previous education in spiritual caring practices assist the nurse in the implementation of spiritual care.

THIS STUDY

The above three factors (the nurse, environment, and educational preparation) provided the background impetus for this present study. It was acknowledged that in looking for 'snapshots' of spiritual caring, entry into a hospice setting was required. Within the hospice setting issues to do with spirituality were more likely to be evident and therefore more able to be identified. In addition, within a palliative care setting, two considerations needed to be acknowledged. Firstly the patient is cared for by a variety of health care professionals (not only the nurse) and secondly, care is given in the context of the patient's family (however defined).

Given the emphasis on 'Educational Preparation' of health care providers expressed in the previous model (Figure 1), entry into any setting would mean discussion (via interview) with these providers, and would assist in determining any educational input required. Therefore, 'interview' was considered an important method for any future study.

AIM OF THIS STUDY

The overall aim of this study therefore was: *To develop a better understanding of spiritual caring in relation to a previous masters' model.* To reach this aim, the main research question generated was:

> From the perspective of the nurse and other health care providers, what constitutes spiritual care giving?

METHODOLOGY

'Spirituality' by its nature resists a research approach that attempts to quantify its character. The 'quantitative' or 'positivist' perspective, a perspective that is used in the physical sciences and emerged from philosophy as 'logical positivism' (Gillis & Jackson, 2002), was therefore discounted. Philosophically, 'positivism' operates an approach to inquiry using deductive rules of objectivity and impersonality (both control the researcher bias) and, using statistical analysis, predictable knowledge is the outcome (Gillis & Jackson, 2002). Under this view, reality exists independent of the knower, the person is viewed as the sum of their parts and adapts to an external environment through cause-and-effect relationships.

However, in more recent years, scientists have been challenged to explain phenomena that defy measurement, particularly 'human' phenomena (Streubert & Carpenter, 1999). The philosophical approach underlying the interpretive paradigm values people in their experiences so that research questions involve human consciousness and subjectivity (Roberts & Taylor, 2002). Further, there is no intent to 'control' the researcher's bias. They are accepted as part of both the research process and the product (Oiler Boyd, 2001).

The qualitative paradigm with its two streams–interpretive and critical (Allen, Benner, & Diekelmann, 1986)–was considered the best choice. Given the emphasis placed on the 'environment' within the previous model and the need to observe spiritual caring, a research approach that acknowledged the setting appeared crucial in any future study. 'Ethnography' (to be discussed) from qualitative *interpretive* research is a methodology that includes the setting in its approach. The interpretive approach refers to the way people 'interpret' the world, giving meaning to events and things. Unlike quantitative approaches where statistical methods are used to investigate the results of the survey and give no information about the context within which the survey is conducted, *interpretive* qualitative research places the interpretive process at the centre of its practice (Rice & Ezzy, 1999, p. 3). People and the meaning they give to things are examined in context.

In selecting a qualitative approach, the 'critical' paradigm was discounted as its emphasis on 'power relations' and evidence of 'emancipation' or change as an outcome (Roberts & Taylor, 2002) was not the focus of the study. Interpretive research is more concerned with description, seeking meaning and gaining understanding of another's world.

Ethnography

From the many qualitative *interpretive* approaches possible (Denzin & Lincoln, 1994), ethnography, which arose from anthropology and is the oldest of the qualitative approaches (Holloway & Wheeler, 1996) was chosen as the most relevant. Ethnography's focus on the environment would allow entry into the setting with the intent to discover the relevance of a previous model in relation to spiritual care. As Boyle (1994) confirms:

> A central tenet of ethnography is that people's behaviour can be understood only in context; this is, in the process of analysis and abstraction, the ethnographer cannot separate elements of human behavior from their relevant context of meaning and purpose. (1994, p. 162)

By entering the setting and interviewing respondents, the meaning of spirituality and spiritual care practices for these respondents would become evident. Using participant observation, ethnography allows for any differences in perception between the researcher and the respondents to be clarified as they occur (Field & Morse, 1985). Knowledge gained through this holistic approach is contextual, reflexive, emic and etic in nature. 'Emic' in that it is derived from respondents (insiders) view of the experience and 'etic' in that it includes the researcher's (outsiders) perception of that reality (Boyle, 1994; Field & Morse, 1985).

Ethical Issues

Prior to entry into the hospice, an informal telephone call was made to the registered nurse in charge of the ward and director of nursing. This initial contact was followed up by a formal letter to both, outlining the study and seeking support. Following their permission approval was sought and obtained from the ethics committee responsible for the conduct of research undertaken in the hospice.

On two separate occasions, an information session was held at the hospice. Here the study was outlined and volunteers sought. Ten registered nurses volunteered and their expectation was that the researcher would, throughout the nursing shift, closely follow them undertaking nursing duties in an assistant capacity only. Once in the setting, other staff members volunteered for interview. Altogether, 13 interviews from staff were available for analysis. These interviews were from ten registered nurses and one each from a volunteer; bereavement counsellor and medical officer.

Prior to interview, a 'plain language statement' was distributed and written consent obtained. All transcripts were returned to respondents for verification. No respondents changed any of the substance of their initial interview. A change was made to some transcripts to include additional information, which surfaced after respondents had read their transcript and on reflection, believed additional information regarding spiritual care should be included.

Methods

Observations were recorded in field notes and these, together with diary entries and documentation were used to contextualise the setting supporting interview data. Although extensive descriptions of the setting were categorised under 'environment' and recorded in field notes, this paper reports on the overall outcome of the study which was derived from interview data.

Data Analysis

Analysis of qualitative data has long been defended against claims of being 'unscientific,' 'passive,' or 'easy' (Munhall, 2001; Denzin & Lincoln, 1994; Morse, 1994). Morse (1994, p. 25) argues analysis requires astute questioning of the data, a relentless search for answers and an accurate recall. For these reasons analysis began as soon as the first interview had been conducted. Further, as the relevance of a previous model was being determined, the three concepts of that model–*the nurse, environment, and educational preparation*–were used initially, to categorise data. That is, questions were posed when analysing the data. For example, did the interview data give information about spiritual nursing practice (or some other), describe the environment or identify educational practice?

Within this study, principle thematic analysis occurred with the 13 interviews. Many qualitative researchers offer guidelines to assist in the task of organising the data into manageable chunks. Colaizzi (in Valle & King, 1978) presents a phenomenological seven-step approach, Miles and Huberman (1984) include a twelve point guide, Burnard (1991) captures fourteen stages while Leininger (1990) suggests a four phase approach. Leininger's (1990) approach was chosen as it is offered for those working with large volumes of ethnographic data and its simplicity meant it was expedient. Her four phases are as follows.

Phase 1

The beginning phase is where the data is collected from its various sources, analysis begins looking for contextual meanings and condensing into a computer. As previously explained, the process of analysis began as soon as the first interview was recorded and all the data were placed into *The Ethnograph version 4.0* (Seidel, Friese, & Leonard, 1995). This computer program arranges the data by single spacing and numbering each line, placing the data in a set format ready for analysis. The program assists in the retrieval of data only; analysis is undertaken by the researcher.

Phase 2

Data are coded and classified as related to the domain of inquiry. Confirming information and establishing credibility and accuracy are of major importance (Leininger, 1990, p. 50).

Confirming information meant analysis began by placing the data into broad categories, i.e., whether the interview data reflected information from patients, staff, relatives, or the researcher. This step was undertaken so the data source could be established and, as the aim was to develop a better understanding of spiritual care, representations (themes) of spiritual care recorded in either words or concepts throughout the transcriptions were noted.

As this step proceeded, unexpected constructs (themes) emerged over and above the initial three categories of the *nurse*, the *environment* and *education*. For example, the major thread *their space* (to be discussed) became obvious soon after data analysis was underway. In any block of discourse (i.e., interview) words that expressed respondent's views of spiritual caring were given a name (code). For example the following extract from interview identifies 3 codes:

> *Researcher:* This morning we were talking about spiritual care. . . .

> *Respondent:* . . . the best approach, the only approach is to listen and learn from them. To find out where they are and then approach it from where they are . . . rather than having some preconceived idea. . . . (No. 5:6-7, 23-28)

Overall, within context, this respondent was replying to my question regarding spiritual caring. Therefore this section of transcript was coded as 'spiritual care.' Further, her own view was to listen (hence the code 'listen') and enter the space of the 'other' (thus the code 'their space). The *Ethnography* computer program allows for this 'layering' of several themes over each other. In this way interviews were read and coded initially over an intense four week period. Interviews were later re-read in light of fresh insights (themes arising from other interviews coded or further insights from field notes or diary entries) and re-coded to include these subsequent themes.

Phase 3

Data are scrutinised to discover saturation of ideas and recurrent patterns of similar or different meanings. The researcher looks for saturation, consistencies, and credibility of data (Leininger, 1990 p. 50). Throughout the research this phase tended to overlap with the second. Following classification of the data into 'codes,' after several re-readings of the text, it became clear that saturation (where no new concepts emerge) had been reached. That is, all the data could be classified into various codes and was then ready for grouping into categories. The categories were: *environment, spiritual care views from staff,* and *spiritual care views from patients.* (This paper reports on staff views of spiritual care only.)

Phase 4

According to Leininger (1990), synthesis and interpretation is the highest phase of data analysis. This phase requires synthesis of thinking, configuration modeling and creative analysis of data from previous phases. The researcher abstracts major themes and findings and may offer theoretical formulations and recommendations (Leininger, 1990).

Even though there were a number of individual themes, within this final phase it was still possible to extract the major focus of the study– *their space.* This concept applied across all interviews of staff and prompted the reconfiguration of the previous model into a new model of spiritual caring. This new model will be presented after the following results section, where extracts from interview are offered to give readers understanding of how it was derived.

RESULTS AND DISCUSSION

The main theme what is termed *their space* emanated from the data. According to Aamodt (1989) a 'cultural theme' is a constant or recurring message (linguistic expression) within ethnography that represents the organising principles in the cultural system under study (Aamodt, 1989, p. 35).

When it came to *spiritual caring*, following discussion with registered nurses, a medical officer, volunteers and bereavement counsellor, all expressed the same sentiment. That is, when spirituality caring for the other, they entered their world, to determine the other's needs.

Ten Registered Nurses' Responses

Lois: . . . *the only approach really is to listen and learn from them. To find out where they are . . . rather than wanting to have some preconceived idea of how they should be coping with death. . . .* (No. 5:24-32)

Sharon: *You have to try and connect with their feelings. What I felt was not important, what was important was what they felt. My feelings had to go down their road.* (No. m 6b:50-67)

Mona: *I usually just listen and ask a few questions . . . it's worth finding out what people do mean by what language they're using . . . it just gives you a few clues . . . as to where they're coming from. . . .* (No. 20:545-555).

Jenny: . . . *I'll ask them how they're seeing it. How they're relating.* (No. 1:49-52)

Mark: . . . *just trying to relate in a relaxed way . . . get to know the patient and adapt to the way they like to do things. . . .* (No. 19:271-275)

Wanda: *It's her beliefs not mine that are important to her . . . to help her to die the way she wanted to. . . .* (No. 14:105-109)

Emily: *I really try to look at individuals. . . . I try to join in with them, even though that is foreign to me. . . .* (No. 18:888-893)

Carol: *It's giving people permission to be themselves. Feeling free to express how they're feeling . . . to be themselves.* (No. 17:48-50).

Rachel: . . . *I think it's being sensitive to each person's spiritual centre, whatever that may be . . . help them to find their peace.* . . . (No. 11:69-72)

Frances: . . . *you just pick up on each patient's individual needs . . . you start to reach a relationship . . . you know what they like.* . . . (No. 15:284-285)

A Medical Officer's Response

Rhonda: *In a sick state they feel very motivated to start looking for answers. But often those answers are other people's answers and they may not be the person's answers.* . . . (No. 8:303-307)

A Volunteer's Response

Sheryl: *Mostly . . . speak gently and follow the patient's line of conversation.* (No. 13:880-883)

A Bereavement Counsellor's Response

James: *But it isn't a kind of them and us. We do this together and we do this in the same safe space.* . . . (No. 9:532-534).

The above expressions enabled a reconceptualising of the original model. The space immediately surrounding the patient (*their space*) is entered into by a variety of health care professionals when offering care. The patient (and their family/significant other) is the centre of care, not the nurse. Within this setting, all health care providers contributed to spiritual care giving and, because of their willingness to offer spiritual care, their education (in spiritual care giving) seemed of limited importance. Consequently, the concepts 'nurse' and 'education' were collapsed into the 'environment' which was described as a 'family' by respondents.

NEW MODEL OF CARE

In this model of care, the centre and main recipient of care is the patient and their family. Surrounding their immediate bed space and identity is a circle, an area called a 'care ring.' On entering *their space*, via the 'care ring,' the nurse or health provider referred to the adaptation they made in their caring, as they accommodated the world of the other. What is claimed as 'spiritual caring' in this study, relates to the preparedness of the health care provider to accommodating the *others* world, in their care. In this way they engaged with their patients, rather than separated from them (see Figure 2).

In determining the other's needs they entered into a dialectic, 'the process of reasoning to obtain truth and knowledge on any topic' (Blackburn, 1996, p. 104). From the registered nursing staff, the ability to determine the patient's needs within this relationship was enhanced by the pattern of nursing care in the ward. Primary nursing, as a way of organising the nursing team, centralises the nurse-patient relationship by linking one patient with one nurse (Bowers, 1989; Manthey, 1973). As a patient's primary nurse, there was more opportunity to engage in the dialectic. It was noted that all health care providers *generally*, referred to the setting as 'family.' For other health care providers, the ability to spend time with the patient was also supported by primary nursing. The principal nurse taking carriage of the patient's care was

FIGURE 2. New Model of Spiritual Care

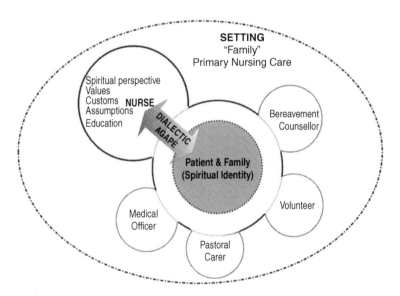

obvious to all health professionals and thus enhanced both individual and collective communication.

Agapé

In claiming the act of entering into another's world as *spiritual,* I would draw parallels with the notion of 'tender loving care' (TLC). A new term for TLC is offered–*agapé.* Agapé expressed here, however, is more than just 'loving care.' It is spiritually connecting with patients sacrificially. Although 'sacrificial giving' is seen as spiritual caring from a Christian perspective, whether or not the patient/client and their relatives express a Christian view of the world, adoption of the underpinning ethos of agapé is surely a behaviour that all health care providers should emulate. When it comes to 'other' centred-ness (what is claimed to be agapé or spiritual caring), encouragement to provide such care is becoming more obvious in the literature. Stickley and Freshwater (2002) argue: "Agapé can be aligned with altruistic love, in which the individual can care for a complete stranger, as if that stranger were family" (2002, p. 251). Other authors support this approach (Watson, 1998), with Fitzgerald (1998) asking "is it possible for caring to be an expression of human agapé in the 21st century?" (1998, p. 32).

It is acknowledged this type of caring can be disarming, particularly when the notion of 'love' is the Western world could be misunderstood as sexual desire. However, a return to the Greek origins of the word brings some clarity. Interpreted in English as a single word 'love,' the Greek language finds three words: 'eros' (erotical, sexual love), 'phileo' (love of friends and family), and 'agapé' (unconditional love), love that seeks the welfare of others. It is this latter concept of agapé that it is suggested is spiritual caring. That is, love that seeks the welfare of others and is not drawn out by any desire in its object, classed as unselfish love, ready to serve (Kittel, Friedrich, & Bromiley, 1995).

Further, given that the model defines spiritual caring as engaging in a dialogue with the patient, interventions termed 'spiritual' may include engaging in discussion around issues of life's meaning, strength or hope in illness. Spiritual care might further include 'affirming, honouring, cherishing, nurturing, and empathetic understanding of the whole person and not just the part' (Cressey & Winbolt-Lewis, 2000, p. 171). Only as concern for others (other conscious) becomes greater than concern for self (self-conscious) will spiritual care be implemented.

CONCLUSION

Given the difficulty with the definition of 'spirituality,' this research began in an attempt to determine spiritual caring from the perspective of nursing staff and other health care providers. It was found that when spiritual caring takes place, nurses and health care providers enter into the space of the other, to determine needs and provide care. In searching for clues the health provider adapts to the world of the other. It is argued this adaptation is spiritual in its nature in that it can be aligned with altruistic love. Here the individual can offer care for a complete stranger, as if that stranger were family (Stickley & Freshwater, 2002).

In illustrating (via a model) the spiritual connection health care providers offer, it is hoped to explicate again the essence of this care. When patients feel health care providers have an interest in their welfare (to the extent the care providers are prepared to put their own values and beliefs aside as they accommodate the other) then–from this research– spiritual care can be seen to be implemented.

REFERENCES

Aamodt, A. M. (1989). Ethnography and Epistemology: Generating nursing knowledge. In Morse, J. M. (Ed.). *Qualitative nursing research. A contemporary dialogue.* Maryland, USA: Aspen Publications Inc.

Allen, D., Benner, P., & Diekelmann, N. (1986). Three paradigms for nursing research: Methodological implications. In P. Chinn (Ed.). *Nursing research methodology: Issues and implementation.* Maryland: Aspen Publishers Inc.

Baldacchino, D., & Draper, P. (2001). Spiritual coping strategies: A review of the nursing research literature. *Journal of Advanced Nursing, 34, 6,* 833-841.

Blackburn, S. (1996). *Oxford dictionary of philosophy.* Oxford: Oxford University Press.

Bolmsjo, I. (2000). Existential issues in palliative care–Interviews with cancer patients. *Journal of Palliative Care, 16,* 20.24.

Bowers, L. (1989). The significance of primary nursing. *Journal of Advanced Nursing, 14, 1,* 13-19.

Bown, J., & Williams, A. (1993). Spirituality and nursing: A review of the literature. *Journal of Advances in Health & Nursing Care, 2, 4,* 41-66.

Boyle, J. (1994). Styles of ethnography. In J. M. Morse (Ed.). *Critical issues in qualitative research methods.* Thousand Oaks, CA: Sage Publications.

Bradshaw, A. (1997). Teaching spiritual care to nurses: An alternative approach. *International Journal of Palliative Care, 3, 1,* 51-57.

Brittain, J. (1986). Theological foundations for spiritual care. *Journal of Religion & Health, 25, 2,* 107-121.

Burnard, P. (1991). A method of analysing interview transcripts in qualitative research. *Nurse Education Today, 11, 6,* 461-466.

Byrne, M. (1999). Editorial–A humbler approach to the unknowable? *Progress in Palliative Care, 7, 1,* 1-2.

Colaizzi, P. (1978). Psychological research as the phenomenologist views it. In R.S. Valle & M. King, (Eds.). *Existential-phenomenological alternatives for psychology.* New York: Oxford University Press.

Cressey, R. W., & Winbolt-Lewis, M. (2000). The forgotten heart of care: A model of spiritual care in the National Health Service. *Accident & Emergency Nursing, 8,* 170-177.

Denzin, N., & Lincoln, Y. (1994). *Handbook of qualitative research* (1st ed). Thousand Oaks, CA: Sage Publications.

Draper, P., & McSherry, W. (2002). A critical view of spirituality and spiritual assessment. *Journal of Advanced Nursing, 39, 1,* 1-2.

Dyson, J., Cobb, M., & Forman, D. (1997). The meaning of spirituality: A literature review. *Journal of Advanced Nursing, 26,* 1183-1188.

Ellis, D. (1980). Whatever happened to the spiritual dimension? *The Canadian Nurse, 76, September,* 42-43.

Emblen, J. (1992). Religion and spirituality defined according to current use in the nursing literature. *Journal of Professional Nursing, 8, 1, January-February,* 41-47.

Emblen, J. D., & Halstead L. (1993). Spiritual needs and interventions: Comparing the views of patients, nurses, and chaplains. *Clinical Nurse Specialist, 7, 4,* 175-182.

Fahlberg, L. L., & Fahlberg, L. A. (1991). Exploring spirituality and consciousness with an expanded science: Beyond the ego with empiricism, phenomenology, and contemplation. *American Journal of Health Promotion, 5, 4,* 273-280.

Field, P., & Morse, J. (1985). *Nursing research–The application of qualitative approaches.* Rockville: Aspen Publishers Inc.

Fitzgerald, L. (1998). Is it possible for caring to be an expression of human agape in the 21st century? *International Journal of Human caring, 2, 3,* 32-39.

Froggatt, K. (1997). Signposts on the journey: The place of ritual in spiritual care. *International Journal of Palliative Care Nursing, 3, 1,* 42-46.

Fry, A., & Tan, L. (1996). The spiritual dimension: Its importance to the nursing care of older people. *Geriaction, 14, 4,* 14-17.

Fryback, P. B., & Reinert, B. R. (1999). Spirituality and people with potentially fatal diagnoses. *Nursing Forum, 34, 1,* 13-22.

Gillis, A., & Jackson, W. (2002). *Research for nurses. Methods and interpretation.* Philadelphia: FA Davis Company.

Grenz, S. J. (1996). *A primer on postmodernism.* Grand Rapids, MI: William. B. Eerdmans Publishing Co.

Groer, M., O'Connor, B., & Droppleman, P. (1996). A course in health care spirituality. *Journal of Nursing Education, 35, 8,* 375-377.

Hamilton, D. G. (1998). Believing in patients' beliefs: Physician attunement to the spiritual dimension as a positive factor in patient healing and health. *The American Journal of Hospice & Palliative Care, September/October*, 276-279.

Harrington, A. (2003). *Spiritual caring in a hospice setting. An ethnography informed by Gadamer's Hermeneutics*. A thesis submitted for the degree of Doctor of Philosophy in the School of Nursing & Midwifery, Flinders University, Adelaide, Australia.

Harrington, A. (1995). Spiritual care: What does it mean to RNs? *Australian Journal of Advanced Nursing, 12, 4*, 5-14.

Harrington, A. (1993). *Registered nurses perceptions of spiritual care. A descriptive study*. Masters Thesis. The Flinders University of South Australia.

Harrison, J. (1993). Spirituality and nursing practice. *Journal of Clinical Nursing, 2*, 211-217.

Holloway, I., & Wheeler, S. (1996). *Qualitative research for nurses*. Oxford: Blackwell Science.

Johnston-Taylor, E., Highfield, M., & Amenta, M. (1994). Attitudes and beliefs regarding spiritual care. *Cancer Nursing, 17, 6*, 479-487.

Kittel, G., Friedrich, G., & Bromiley, G. (1995). *Theological dictionary of the New Testament*. Grand Rapids, MI: WB Eerdmans.

Leininger, M. (1990). Ethnomethods: The philosophic and epistemic bases to explicate transcultural nursing knowledge. *Journal of Transcultural Nursing, 1, 2*, 40-51.

McSherry, W. (2000). Education issues surrounding the teaching of spirituality. *Nursing Standard, 14, 42*, 40-43.

McSherry, W., & Draper, P. (1998). The debates emerging from the literature surrounding the concept of spirituality as applied to nursing. *Journal of Advanced Nursing, 27*, 683-691.

Manthey, M. (1973). Primary Nursing is alive and well in the hospital. *American Journal of Nursing, 73(1)*, 83-87.

Mickley, J. R., Soeken, K., & Belcher, A. (1992). Spiritual well-being, religiousness, and hope among women with breast cancer. *IMAGE: Journal of Nursing Scholarship, 24, 4*, 267-272.

Miles, M., & Huberman, A. (1984). *Qualitative data analysis. A sourcebook of new methods*. Beverly Hills, CA: Sage Publications.

Morse, J. (1994). Emerging from the data: The cognitive processes of analysis in qualitative inquiry. In J. M. Morse (Ed.). *Critical issues in qualitative research methods*. Thousand Oaks, CA: Sage Publications.

Munhall, P. (2001). Language and nursing research. In P. L. Munhall & C. Oiler Boyd (Eds.). *Nursing research: A qualitative perspective* (3rd ed). National League for Nursing, Sudbury, USA: Jones and Barlett.

Narayanasamy, A. (1999). A review of spirituality as applied to nursing. *International Journal of Nursing Studies, 36*, 117-125.

Oiler Boyd, C. (2001). Philosophical foundations of qualitative research. In P. L. Munhall & C. Oiler Boyd (Eds.). *Nursing research: A qualitative perspective* (3rd ed). National League for Nursing, MA: Jones and Bartlett.

Oldnall, A. (1996). A critical analysis of nursing: Meeting the spiritual needs of patients. *Journal of advanced Nursing, 23*, 138-144.

Relf, M. V. (1997). Illuminating meaning and transforming issues of spirituality in HIV disease and AIDS: An application of Parse's theory of human becoming. *Holistic Nursing Practice, 12, 1*, 1-8.

Rice, P., & Ezzy, D. (1999). *Qualitative research methods. A health focus.* South Melbourne, Victoria: Oxford University Press.

Roberts, K., & Taylor B. (2002). *Nursing research processes. An Australian perspective* (2nd ed). Victoria: Nelson, (Thomson Learning).

Ross, L. (1994). The spiritual dimension: Its importance to patients' health, well-being, and quality of life and its implications for nursing practice. *International Journal of Nursing Studies, 32, 5*, 457-468.

Seidel, J., Friese, S., & Leonard, D. (1995). *The ethnograph v.4: A Users Guide.* Boulder CO: Waiting Room Press.

Smith, J., & McSherry, W. (2004). Spirituality and child development: A concept analysis. *Journal of Advanced Nursing, 45, 3*, 307-315.

Stickley, T., & Freshwater, D. (2002). The art of loving and the therapeutic relationship. *Nursing Inquiry, 9, 4*, 250-256.

Streubert, H., & Carpenter, D. (1999). *Qualitative research in nursing. Advancing the hermanistic imperative* (2nd ed). Philadelphia: Lippincott, Williams & Wilkins.

Watson, J. (1998). A meta reflection on reflective practice and caring theory. In C. Johns & D. Freshwater (Eds.). *Transforming nursing through reflective practice.* Oxford: Blackwell Science.

PART II

A Palliative Approach to Spirituality in Residential Aged Care

Linda Kristjanson, RN, BN, MN, PhD

SUMMARY. This paper describes how a palliative approach to care is relevant in the context of residential aged care, with specific focus on the spiritual needs of residents. Three issues are described that make attention to spirituality in residential aged care particularly challenging: effects of cognitive changes, potential threats to dignity, and uncertainties about how to provide bereavement support to the range of people who experience loss in this care context. Reflections on how residential aged care staff might better assess the spiritual needs of residents are offered with suggestions from the literature about how to sensitively respond to these needs. *[Article copies available for a fee from The Haworth Document Delivery Service: 1-800-HAWORTH. E-mail address: <docdelivery@haworthpress. com> Website: <http://www.HaworthPress.com> © 2006 by The Haworth Press, Inc. All rights reserved.]*

KEYWORDS. Palliative care, spirituality, aged care, dignity, bereavement, cognitive impairment

---

Linda Kristjanson, RN, BN, MN, PhD, is The Cancer Council WA Chair of Palliative Care, WA Centre for Cancer & Palliative Care, Edith Cowan University, Pearson Street, Churchlands, WA 6018, Australia (E-mail: L.Kristjanson@ecu.eu.au).

[Haworth co-indexing entry note]: "A Palliative Approach to Spirituality in Residential Aged Care." Kristjanson, Linda. Co-published simultaneously in *Journal of Religion, Spirituality & Aging* (The Haworth Pastoral Press, an imprint of The Haworth Press, Inc.) Vol. 18, No. 4, 2006, pp. 189-205; and: *Aging, Spirituality and Palliative Care* (ed: Elizabeth MacKinlay) The Haworth Pastoral Press, an imprint of The Haworth Press, Inc., 2006, pp. 189-205. Single or multiple copies of this article are available for a fee from The Haworth Document Delivery Service [1-800-HAWORTH, 9:00 a.m. - 5:00 p.m. (EST). E-mail address: docdelivery@haworthpress.com].

This paper will provide a brief description of the term "a palliative approach to care" and outline why this approach is important to residential aged care and the spiritual needs of this group of people. The paper will then examine three key issues that make attention to spirituality in residential aged care particularly challenging: the effects of cognitive changes, potential threats to dignity, and uncertainties about how to provide bereavement support to the range of people who experience loss in this care context. And finally, this paper concludes by offering some reflections on how residential aged care staff might better address the spiritual needs of individuals in residential aged care facilities and their families from the perspective of a palliative approach.

WHAT IS A PALLIATIVE APPROACH?

A palliative approach aims to improve the quality of life for individuals with a life-limiting illness and their families, by reducing their suffering through early identification, assessment, and treatment of pain, physical, cultural, psychological, social, and spiritual needs (Kristjanson et al., 2003).

Underlying the philosophy of a palliative approach is a positive and open attitude towards death and dying. The promotion of a more open approach to discussions of death and dying between the aged care team, residents, and their families facilitates identification of their wishes regarding end-of-life care. A palliative approach is not confined to the end stages of an illness. Instead, a palliative approach provides a focus on active comfort care and a positive approach to reducing an individual's symptoms and distress, which facilitates residents' and their families' understanding that they are being actively supported through this process (Kristjanson et al., 2003).

The World Health Organisation (2002) defines palliative care as:

> An approach that improves the quality of life of individuals and their families facing the problem associated with life-threatening illness, through the prevention and relief of suffering by means of early identification and impeccable assessment and treatment of pain and other problems, physical, psychosocial, and spiritual.

This recent definition and description of palliative care asserts that, contrary to earlier definitions of palliative care, individuals with diseases other than cancer that have a terminal phase and are progressive in nature would benefit from the philosophical underpinning of the palliative approach. However, there are other incurable diseases that are equally as debilitating and that necessitate a palliative approach in their terminal stages, such as Chronic Obstructive Pulmonary Disease (COPD), Alzheimer's disease, and acute massive cerebrovascular accidents.

The definition also states that to provide a palliative approach, the health team must provide an impeccable assessment and treatment of pain and other problems, physical, psychosocial, and spiritual. The importance of assessing the spiritual needs of individuals receiving a palliative approach and the salience of responding appropriately to these needs is clearly evident in this definition. How do we undertake a spiritual assessment and how do we best respond? What are the particular issues that must be addressed in the context of spiritual support to older individuals in a palliative phase of an illness? These questions will be addressed in this paper.

THE NEED FOR A PALLIATIVE APPROACH IN RESIDENTIAL AGED CARE

In Australia, over the last two decades, research has indicated that the proportion of people dying in residential aged care facilities (RACFs) has steadily increased (Giles et al., 2003). The increased number of residents dying in RACFs has led to the recognition that a palliative approach enhances the care already provided to both residents and their families (DeBellis & Parker, 1998; Keay, 1999).

The unique setting of RACFs and the diverse profile of their residents create significant difficulties in using a palliative approach. Not only do the majority of residents have dementia; they generally have co-morbidities (other diseases) that involve physical, psychological, emotional, and social boundaries. The residents are generally highly dependent and require many medications, further complicating the provision of a palliative approach.

The Australian Palliative Residential Aged Care (APRAC) Project (2002) was established in response to recognition that there was a critical need for a palliative approach in residential aged care. The project consisted of three components:

- Development of national guidelines for a palliative approach in residential aged care.

- Development of a national education and training program to ensure that all residential aged care staff are able to access suitable training to facilitate the provision of a palliative approach.
- Identification of options for communication and implementation of the guidelines and the education and training program.

The information gained from this study revealed specific issues that make provision of spiritual palliative support particularly challenging in the context of residential aged care facilities.

A PALLIATIVE APPROACH IN RESIDENTIAL AGED CARE

People entering RACFs are increasingly frail. Authors of a recent Australian study projected a 70% increase over the next 30 years of the number of older persons with profound disabilities, particularly for those aged 65 years or older (Giles et al., 2003). The main conditions for older persons with profound disability are neurological, musculoskeletal, circulatory and respiratory. Stroke also severely debilitates. Mild to moderate disabilities are associated with poor vision and hearing, psychiatric disorders and cancer. Residents are likely to have more than one of these disabilities and their management is likely to be complex due to the existence of co-morbidities. These disabilities significantly contribute to restrictions in daily activities such as self-care, mobility, and communication.

A significant increase in the number of individuals aged 75 to 94 years with a profound restriction is also projected to occur from 2011 to 2021 (Giles et al., 2003). This increase is anticipated to have major implications for care delivery.

THREE FORMS OF PALLIATIVE CARE

In considering palliative care for residents in RACFs, it is important to distinguish amongst a palliative approach, specialised palliative care service provision, and end-of-life or terminal care (Kristjanson et al., 2003). The distinction among these forms of palliative care is important in care planning and clarifying the goals for treatment for residents.

A Palliative Approach

When the resident's condition is not amenable to cure and the symptoms of the disease require effective symptom management, a palliative approach is appropriate. Provision of active treatment for the resident's disease may also still be important and may be provided concurrently with a palliative approach. However, the primary goal of a palliative approach is to improve a resident's level of comfort and function, and to address his/her psychological/spiritual/social requirements.

Specialised Palliative Service Provision

This form of palliative care involves referral to a specialised palliative team or health care practitioner. However, this form of palliative care does not replace a palliative approach. Rather, involvement of a specialised palliative service augments a palliative approach with focused, intermittent specific input as required. The goals are the assessment and treatment of complex symptoms experienced by the resident and provision of information and advice that is related to complex issues (e.g., ethical dilemmas, family issues, or psychological or existential distress) for the aged care team.

End-of-Life (Terminal) Care

This form of palliative care is appropriate when the resident is in the final days or weeks of life and care decisions may need to be reviewed more frequently. Goals are more sharply focused on the resident's physical, emotional, and spiritual comfort and support for the family.

SPIRITUALITY IN RESIDENTIAL AGED CARE

Spiritual care should be an essential part of comprehensive residential aged care, but is probably the least understood and most often neglected aspect of care (Cobb, 2001). According to Woodruff (2004), every person, be they religious or not, possesses a unique form of spirituality. Spirituality encompasses the purpose and meaning of an individual's existence and involves relationships with and perceptions of people and all other things and events. Spirituality is founded in cultural, religious, and family traditions, and is modified by life experiences (Woodruff, 2004).

Spiritual beliefs, whether or not associated with religious practice, contain tenets about the course of human life and existence beyond it (Walsh et al., 2002). Impending death or the death of a close relative or companion is an extremely distressing experience and spiritual questions and concerns may become particularly palpable at these times.

In the context of residential aged care, the challenges of providing spiritual support can be considerable. Three broad challenges are particularly unique to this group: cognitive changes, potential for loss of dignity, and uncertainties of how to provide bereavement support in this care context.

Cognitive Changes

According to a recent report, more than 162,000 Australians had dementia in 2002, and it is anticipated that 500,000 people will have dementia by the year 2040 (Giles et al., 2003). Dementia is currently the second largest cause of disability in Australia (depression is the first) and by 2016 dementia is expected to be the primary cause of major chronic illness (Giles et al., 2003). Approximately half of the people diagnosed with dementia live in a RACF (Gibson et al., 1999).

Overall, 30% of residents in low care facilities and approximately 60% of residents in high care facilities have dementia. Only 10% of high care residents have no cognitive impairment (Gibson et al., 1999). However, this data is based upon a documented diagnosis, suggesting that these figures are likely under-estimates of the prevalence of the condition.

Advanced dementia is a neurological disease characterised by severe cognitive decline of an irreversible nature that is associated with poor prognostic factors such as swallowing disturbance, weight loss, dysphagia, anorexia, bowel and bladder incontinence, often resulting in the person being bedridden (Ahronheim et al., 2000). Advanced dementia is also known as late stage or severe dementia. The progression from diagnosis of advanced dementia to death is usually three years (Hurley et al., 1993). Poorer prognosis is likely if the resident develops an acute illness such as pneumonia (van der Steen et al., 2002) or an infectious disease (Hurley et al., 1993). Thus, advanced dementia is a progressive degenerative disease that is life limiting and a palliative approach to care should be offered (Hurley et al., 1993).

There is evidence to suggest that a palliative approach benefits not only the individual with the disease, but also the family (Casarett et al., 2002). The features of a palliative approach considered most helpful to the family are continual follow-up evaluation, attention to all symptoms causing distress, emphasis on the resident's quality of life, attention to the resident's sense of dignity and avoidance of hospitalisation whenever possible (Casarett et al., 2002). Underlying a palliative approach is the assumption that all residents with advanced dementia should be thoroughly assessed with a view to managing all treatable causes of confusion.

The fact of cognitive impairment calls into question the whole area of spirituality. Is cognitive function necessary for a spiritual life? How does a change in cognitive awareness affect spirituality? How does a loss of cognitive capacity affect communication about spiritual issues? How important is memory to spirituality?

There is no doubt that communication about spirituality is challenged by changes in an individual's cognitive abilities and illuminate the extent to which many of our "therapies" or care interventions are "talk based," relying upon a polite and logical interchange of ideas. Communication with someone with cognitive dementia may not be logical or follow the usual social scripts. However, if Watzlawick's (1967) classic communication theory is correct, and there is "no such thing as not communicating" and at least 80% of communication is nonverbal, communication need not rely on logical, sequential, verbal exchange. Communication with someone who is cognitively impaired regarding any matter, including spirituality, is therefore theoretically possible. It might also be imagined that communication related to spirituality with someone who is cognitively impaired might be enhanced, because usual social conformities related to how to discuss religion and beliefs may be less dominant, allowing more authentic communication between two people. The ways to assess a person's spiritual needs and support their spiritual needs may need to be less verbal, more symbolic and more creative.

Dignity

In the context of a palliative approach, promotion of an individual's sense of dignity is a central touchstone. Dignity is important in the context of spirituality and palliative aged care because a person's sense of dignity is linked very closely to their sense of meaning and quality of life. Residents in aged care facilities are susceptible to assaults on their sense of dignity and sense of purpose and may become isolated and feel under-valued.

Individuals may hold different views about what dignity means and in the face of a progressive illness or the ageing process, the meaning of dignity may change over time. The aged care team's perception of dignity may differ from the resident's view. The best way to understand what dignity means for an individual resident is to ask each resident and family what are the most important factors for him or her in relation to dignity. The aged care team members who endeavour to respect the dignity of residents need to acknowledge the things that are considered important to the individual in enhancing and maintaining their dignity.

Our research team has worked with a team of colleagues in Canada and Australia to better understand the concept of dignity in the context of a palliative approach (Chochinov et al., 2002a). Our team identified a Dignity-Conserving Care Model for a palliative approach that is aimed at helping the individual to feel valued (Chochinov et al., 2002b). This framework was based upon a series of qualitative studies that helped to identify the central factors that could enhance or diminish a person's sense of dignity. Three broad factors emerged from our work: illness/ageing-related issues, dignity-converting strategies, and a social dignity inventory.

Illness/ageing related concerns are those things that directly result from the illness or ageing progression (e.g., loss of independence, physical symptom distress, changes to cognitive status, functional abilities). Dignity-converting strategies are those influences related to the resident's psychological and spiritual resources. These include two types: dignity preserving perspectives and dignity enhancing practices. Dignity preserving perspectives have to do with the way the person sees themselves, their outlook, their way of making sense of things (e.g., maintenance of pride, sense of generativity/legacy, or a feeling that they are leaving something behind to be remembered by), continuity of self, self-esteem, hopefulness, role preservation, autonomy, acceptance, and resilience.

Dignity conserving practices include things such as prayer, meditation, and taking one day at a time. This work also underscores the importance of the "care tenor" or manner in which residents are treated, reminding the health care provider to be respectful in all communication. The ways in which a person is treated reinforces or diminishes his/her sense of dignity.

Finally, the social dignity inventory includes those environmental and social influences that can affect dignity, such as privacy boundaries, social support, and concerns of being a burden. Patients also talked about aftermath concerns–of worries that they would leave things unfinished or troubled for their loved ones. The fear that they would die without attending to these aftermath concerns was a factor that diminished their sense of dignity.

We have developed and tested an approach to care that is a positive, strength-based reflective interview that aims to bolster the individual's sense of dignity. This intervention consists of having patients speak to those things they would want addressed or documented before dying (Chochinov et al., 2005; McClement et al., 2004). These sessions are tape recorded, transcribed, and then edited so as to transform the dialogue format into a coherent narrative. The resulting 'Generativity Document' is returned to the patient for them to bequeath to their families.

Results from our Phase I trial indicate that this is a highly effective intervention that patients feel increase their preparedness for death, heightens their sense of dignity, increases their will to live, and helps prepare their family for the future (Chochinov et al., 2005). The work has now been funded through a grant from the National Institute of Health to progress this to a randomised clinical trial for people with advanced terminal illness.

We are also embarking upon a study of the dignity interview in the aged care population with a grant from National Health & Medical Research Council (NH&MRC). The purpose of this pilot project is to modify and assess this novel intervention with elderly residents and their family members, to determine the benefits to family members and elderly residents. We will do this using two approaches.

First, we will explore the feasibility of having family and resident participate together in co-constructing a generativity document. We have some experience with this in our pilot work, and found that the process was facilitated by giving family members a sense of constructive involvement. Another format we will pilot involves family members who will construct the generativity document by proxy. There are many instances when the resident is no longer well enough to participate in psychosocial interventions due to fatigue, dementia, or rapid deterioration. In those instances, it will be important to determine whether family members are able to construct generativity documents that capture the resident's essence. Our work has shown that dignity often is dependent on the perception of how one is seen. Therefore, generativity documents will be provided with the residents and family's permission to the residential care team as a 'perception altering strategy,' possibly enhancing their appreciation for the resident.

Any approaches to care that bolster the person's sense of dignity, sense of self-worth, and feelings of purpose and meaning are important to foster and may be a way of enriching the spirit.

Bereavement Support

There is much controversy in the recent literature regarding the merits of various types of bereavement support. Most of this literature has been limited by a lack of sound theoretical frameworks to guide the studies, measurement difficulties, non-comparable study samples, and poorly described dosages and types of bereavement intervention. These flaws have clouded interpretations of bereavement studies. Nonetheless, the issue of bereavement is often closely linked to questions of spirituality, meaning, relationships, loss, hope, loneliness, and uncertainty. Therefore, the health team endeavouring to offer spiritual support at the time of bereavement or simply bereavement support at the time of bereavement finds themselves challenged by how best to help the person navigate the difficult terrain of loss and grief.

A full discussion of bereavement literature is beyond the scope of this paper. However, it is important to note that previous theories of "stages of grief" are now being questioned, and the notion of integrating grief and loss into one's life is becoming a more helpful construct. The individual who is grieving is not asked to "get over it" or " move on"–but is helped to reflect, remember, and move forward, while looking back at the parts of the lost relationship that emerge (Cleiren, 1993; Walter, 1996). Grief is a biological experience as well as an emotional, spiritual and cognitive one. As a result, grief becomes an enduring, sometimes relenting, and sometimes poignant, but always present part of the life of a person who has lost. How do these conceptualisations about grief inform our approach to bereavement in the context of aged care?

Bereavement Support for Other Residents

It is inevitable that residents will witness the death of other residents. The evidence suggests that bereavement support needs of residents are often centred on offering practical and emotional support at these times (Katz et al., 2000). However, some staff in RACFs may be concerned about the impact of a resident's death on those sharing the same room and questions of how to best "protect" the surviving resident may surface.

Despite the expected negative consequences, there can be benefits for other individuals who witness someone else's death. For example, hospice patients who witnessed a fellow patient's death found this awareness of dying to be both comforting and distressing (Payne et al., 1996). The researchers found that those that had witnessed a death were significantly less depressed than those patients who had not had this experience. This finding raises questions therefore about the possible benefits of exposure to death within the residential aged care setting and points to the need for support to help residents come to terms with this type of loss.

Bereavement Support for Residents with Advanced Dementia

The mourning process is not exclusive to those who can cognitively manage the grieving process. Residents with advanced dementia are also affected by grief and loss, but may not have the cognitive skills to resolve or make sense of their grief. A resident's fluctuating lucidity may make it difficult for the aged care team and family to determine what he/she knows, understands or comprehends regarding the death of another resident. Benbow and Quinn (1990) recommend that the aged care team be honest and consistent with residents, allowing them time to grieve even if they forget the details. Protecting residents from the truth can create greater confusion, because the story will not match the reality. Residents with advanced dementia may need bereavement support for an extended length of time before they can accept the reality of the loss.

Bereavement Support for Family Members

Many families also mourn the loss of relationship with the person with advanced dementia and may require support in dealing with this 'double death.' People suffering with dementia have often been termed 'the living dead' and family members, in particular spouses, find the progressive degeneration difficult to watch and the grieving process is often protracted and painful (Anderson et al., 1992). RACFs that have a dementia support group in place where issues of grief and loss are addressed may help provide families with the support they require. One study found that support groups for bereaved seniors enhanced satisfaction with support given, diminished feelings of loneliness and positively increased their emotional affect (Stewart et al., 2001). This study was conducted with widows living by themselves in the community, so the findings whilst pertinent to this discussion might not be applicable to males and younger people (e.g., children of residents). There is a clear need for further research in this area. Additional research is also required to determine the suitability of support groups in communal settings, such as RACFs, to assist residents to cope with the deaths of other residents.

So how do we best offer bereavement support in the context of palliative aged care? We need to acknowledge the many losses, sorrow, and grief that the residents will experience. We need to anticipate that enduring and repeating feelings of loss and grief remain present, and offer focused attention to families, residents, and carers.

Spiritual Support

Spirituality has been found to be an important predictor of the quality of life of individuals receiving a palliative approach (Hermann, 2001; Thomson, 2000). Impending death is considered a powerful stimulus for reflection on the significance of life and destiny for residents in RACFs (Koenig et al., 1997). Therefore, an early assessment of the spiritual needs of residents is important and should not be relegated to a later stage of the illness.

Spiritual assessment is an ongoing process. Understanding the resident's current or desired practices, attitudes, experiences, and beliefs assists in meeting the spiritual needs of residents (Hermann, 2001). The aged care team needs to determine whether a resident embraces some form of spirituality and the ways in which the resident practices this belief. Simply asking a resident which religion he/she belongs to is not an adequate means of determining a resident's spiritual needs. Some suggestions about how the aged care team might begin discussions of spiritual needs are included in the APRAC Guidelines. Possible questions that might be posed include:

- How are you in yourself?
- What is your source of hope and strength?
- What are your spiritual needs?
- Are there ways we might help with your spiritual needs or concerns?

In addition, according to Hicks (1999), things to observe that may reflect spiritual need include:

- Social Isolation;
- Depression;
- Resident questioning meaning of their existence;

- Resident seeking spiritual assistance;
- Resident attendance at spiritual services; and
- Religious items or practices.

Similarly, obtaining a comprehensive social/family history that includes these issues from the resident or family at time of admission may help to identify the resident's own past and present resources for their spiritual care (Hermann, 2001). The evidence suggests that spiritual assessment is best conducted in a trusting environment by a person with adequate interpersonal skills who is able to engage the views of the resident and the family through use of a conversational style rather than a fact-finding interrogation (Hermann, 2001).

A regular review will guide practice, ensuring that spiritual care is flexible and adaptable, meeting the needs of the resident and family, particularly when needs change (e.g., when death is imminent). Whether a resident's spiritual care involves public or private practices, the resident's privacy needs to be respected and an opportunity provided for such practices to continue according to the need (Hermann, 2001; Wilson & Daley, 1999). Spiritual counselling and support are essential to a palliative approach and may help provide rites and rituals that offer symbolic meaning to residents (Orchard & Clark, 2001). Social isolation, questions on the meaning of life, depression, or a search for spiritual assistance may indicate that a resident requires spiritual attention.

Spiritual care involves assisting residents to articulate those things that are important to them personally. Spiritual care involves sensitive listening skills, rather than providing answers. It is not necessary for the aged care team to share the same spiritual beliefs as the resident in order to understand the resident's spiritual needs, nor is the aim of spiritual care for members of the aged care team to impose their own views (McGrath et al., 1999). This care includes an awareness of the feelings of isolation the resident may experience at the end-of-life (McKinlay, 2001). Hicks (1999) identified three key interventions that may be helpful in offering spiritual support to residents: silent support, liaison, and active listening. Silent support includes being with the resident, providing a supportive presence, and being non-judgemental. Liaison refers to coordinating services and individuals requested by the resident (chaplains/pastoral care workers, family, friends), ensuring access to spiritual activities (Bible study, worship ceremonies), obtaining requested spiritually related items (e.g., books, rosaries, statues, videos, music), and avoiding interrupting resident during spiritual activities.

Active listening involves engaging in conversation with the resident, being alert to the resident's comfort level–watch for eye contact, bodily movement (turning away, restlessness), and disengagement from conversation, and repeating themes of the conversation to ensure accurate interpretation.

Chaplains and pastoral care workers can provide spiritual care to people in a variety of settings. The inclusion of either a chaplain or pastoral care worker in an aged care team is advocated in the APRAC guidelines (2002) to facilitate a palliative approach that considers each resident's spiritual care needs.

In a recent UK study, 73% of residential facilities surveyed (N = 1,500) had requested the assistance of someone from the Christian faith to help care for a dying resident (Orchard & Clark, 2001). Fourteen percent had called in support from other faiths, such as Judaism, Baha'ism and Humanism. This external help was requested because 67% of the RACF managers felt that it would benefit the resident. This suggests that the aged care team may perceive increased spiritual needs at the time of death and readily seek assistance from people who are well trained in the area of spirituality. These findings point to the relevance of access to chaplains and pastoral care workers for residents requiring a palliative approach. However, unless the resident wants spiritual support, a visit from a chaplain/pastoral care worker can be considered an intrusion.

Most importantly, to be effective in providing spiritual support, the chaplain/pastoral care worker should have experience and knowledge about spiritual issues and should be an integral part of a multidisciplinary team (Hermann, 2001). However, other members of the aged care team are often asked questions relating to spiritual matters by residents and these are best addressed at the time by the aged care team in an open, non-judgemental manner (Hermann, 2001). Three guidelines related to spiritual care are outlined in the APRAC guidelines (2002):

1. A palliative approach supports residents and families to express their unique spirituality. Respecting their privacy and providing an opportunity for them to continue their spiritual practices enhances a resident's spiritual care and their quality of life, as does spiritual counselling.
2. Understanding the resident's current or desired practices, attitudes, experiences, and beliefs by obtaining a comprehensive history, assists in meeting the spiritual needs of a resident, as does a regular review.

3. The aged care team is encouraged to respond in an open, non-judgemental manner to residents' questions relating to spiritual matters. Involving a chaplain/pastoral care worker with experience and knowledge about these issues is considered best practice.

CONCLUSION

This article has offered some perspectives on a palliative approach in the context of residential aged care and has highlighted some of the key issues that emerge when one considers the spiritual needs of people in this stage of life. Questions about how to respectfully assess the spiritual needs of residents and respond in a helpful way have been explored. The challenges of how to provide spiritual support to individuals with cognitive impairment have been outlined and the importance of promoting a resident's sense of dignity as a fundamental aspect of spiritual care has been discussed. And finally, questions have been posed about how to support the spirit when bereavement occurs and questions of meaning re-emerge.

These questions and challenges are not simple and the answers cannot be offered in a glib or superficial manner. Rather, our capacity to respond to perhaps the most complex and important aspect of a palliative approach in aged care calls upon our humanity and our capacity to remain engaged.

REFERENCES

Ahronheim, J., Morrison, S., Morris, J., Baskin, S. A., & Meier, D. E. (2000). Palliative care in advanced dementia: A randomized controlled trial and descriptive analysis. *Journal of Palliative Medicine, 3, 3,* 265-273.

Anderson, K. H., Hobson, A., Steiner, P., & Rodel, B. (1992). Patients with dementia-involving families to maximise nursing care. *Journal of Gerontological Nursing, 18, 7,* 19-25.

Australian Palliative Residential Aged Care Project (2002). *Palliative care service provision in Australia: A planning guide.* Canberra: Palliative Care Australia.

Benbow, S. M., & Quinn, A. (1990). Dementia, grief, and dying. *Palliative Medicine, 4, 2,* 87-92.

Casarett, D., Takesaka, J., Karlawish, J., Hirschman, K. B., & Clark, C. M. (2002). How should clinicians discuss hospice for patients with dementia? Anticipating caregivers' preconceptions and meeting their information needs. *Alzheimer Disease & Associated Disorders, 16, 2,* 116-122.

Chochinov, H. M., Hack, T., Hassard, T., Kristjanson, L., McClement, S., & Harlos, M. (2002a). *Dignity in the terminally ill: A cross-sectional, cohort study. Lancet, 360 (9350)*, 2026-2030.

Chochinov, H. M., Hack, T., Hassard, T., Kristjanson, L. J., McClement, S., & Harlos, M. (2005). Dignity therapy: A novel psychotherapeutic intervention for patients near the end of life. *Journal of Clinical Oncology, 23* (24), 5520-5525.

Chochinov, H. M., Hack, T., McClement, S., Harlos, M., & Kristjanson, L. J. (2002b). Dignity in the terminally ill: An empirical model. *Social Science & Medicine, 54, 3*, 433-443.

Cleiren, M. (1993). *Bereavement and adaptation. A comparative study of the aftermath of death*. Washington: Hemisphere Publishing.

Cobb, M. (2001). *The dying soul. Spiritual care at the end of life*. Buckingham: Open University Press.

De Bellis, A., & Parker, D. (1998). Providing palliative care in Australian nursing homes: Issues and challenges. *Geriaction, 16, 3*, 17-23.

Gibson, D., Benham, C., & Racic, L. (Eds.). (1999). *Older Australia at a glance* (2nd ed.). Canberra, Australian Capital Territory: Australian Institute of Health and Welfare.

Giles, L. C., Cameron, I. D., & Crotty, M. (2003). Disability in older Australians: Projections for 2006-2031. *Medical Journal of Australia, 179, 3*, 130-133.

Hermann, C. P. (2001). Spiritual needs of dying patients: A qualitative study. *Oncology Nursing Forum, 28, 1*, 67-72.

Hicks, T. J. J. (1999). Spirituality and the elderly: Nursing implications with nursing home residents. *Geriatric Nursing, 20, 3*, 144-146.

Hurley, A., Volicer, B. J., Mahoney, M., & Volicer, L. (1993). Palliative fever management in Alzheimer patients: Quality plus fiscal responsibility. *Advances in Nursing Science, 16, 1*, 21-32.

Katz, J., Sidell, M., & Komaromy, C. (2000). Death in homes: Bereavement needs of residents, relatives and staff. *International Journal of Palliative Nursing, 6, 6*, 274-279.

Keay, T. J. (1999). Palliative care in the nursing home. *Generations, 23, 1*, 96-98.

Koenig, H. G., Weiner, D. K., Peterson, B. L., Meador, K. G., & Keefe, F. J. (1997). Religious coping in the nursing home: A biopsychosocial model. *International Journal of Psychiatry in Medicine, 27, 4*, 365-76.

Kristjanson, L. J., Toye, C. T., & Dawson, S. (2003). New dimensions in palliative care: A palliative approach to neurodegenerative diseases and final illness in older people. *Medical Journal of Australia, 179, Suppl. 6*, S42-44.

McClement, S. E., Chochinov, H. M., Hack, T. F., Kristjanson, L.J., & Harlos, M. (2004). Dignity-conserving care: Application of research findings into practice. *International Journal of Palliative Nursing, 10, 4*, 173-179.

McGrath, P., Yates, P., Clinton, M., & Hart, G. (1999). "What should I say?": Qualitative findings on dilemmas in palliative care nursing. *Hospice Journal, 14, 2*, 17-33.

McKinlay, E. M. (2001). Within the circle of care: Patient experiences of receiving palliative care. *Journal of Palliative Care, 17, 1*, 22-29.

Orchard, H., & Clark, D. (2001). Tending the soul as well as the body: Spiritual care in nursing and residential homes. *International Journal of Palliative Nursing, 7, 11*, 541-546.

Payne, S., Hillier, R., Langley-Evans, A., & Roberts, T. (1996). Impact of witnessing death on hospice patients. *Social Science & Medicine, 43, 12,* 1785-94.

Stewart, M., Craig, D., MacPherson, K., & Alexander, S. (2001). Promoting positive affect and diminishing loneliness of widowed seniors through a support intervention. *Public Health Nursing, 18, 1,* 54-63.

Thomson, J. E. (2000). The place of spiritual well-being in hospice patient's overall quality of life. *Hospice Journal, 15, 2,* 13-27.

Van der Steen, J. T., Ooms, M. E., Mehr, D. R., Van der Wal, G., & Ribbe, M. W. (2002). Severe dementia and adverse outcomes of nursing home-acquired pneumonia: Evidence for mediation by functional and pathophysiological decline. *Journal of the American Geriatrics Society, 50, 3,* 439-448.

Walsh, K., Jones, L., Tookman, A., & Blizard, R. (2002). Spiritual beliefs may affect outcome of bereavement: Prospective study. *British Medical Journal, 324, 7353,* 1551-1560.

Walter, T. (1996). A new model of grief: Bereavement and biography. *Mortality, 1, 1,* 7-25.

Watzlawick, C. (1967). *Pragmatics of human communication.* New York: Norton.

Wilson, S. A., & Daley, B. J. (1999). Family perspectives on dying in long-term care settings. *Journal of Gerontological Nursing, 25, 11,* 19-25.

Woodruff, R., (2004). *Palliative medicine: Evidence-based symptomatic and supportive care for patients with advanced cancer* (4th ed). New York: Oxford University Press.

World Health Organization (2002). *National cancer control programmes: Policies and managerial guidelines* (2nd ed.). Geneva: WHO.

Learning to Be a Professional:
Two Models of Competence
and Related Learning Strategies

Laurie Grealish, RN, MN, Oncology Certificate, FRCNA

SUMMARY. Occupations required by the health industry, specifically in aged and palliative care, include nursing, pastoral care, medicine, and social work amongst many others. Professional education for these health disciplines incorporates competence for practice and critical thinking skills. Two different conceptual models of competence, personal and operational, reveal different approaches to learning. Personal competence, currently dominant in the higher eduction (tertiary) sector, privileges theory over practice. Personal competence can exclude non-propositional forms of knowledge, making it difficult for students to explain their practice experiences. The operational model of competence, which is emerging in professional education, has the potential to develop critical approaches to learning and practice, skills required for practice development and quality improvement in today's health environment. *[Article copies available for a fee from The Haworth Document Delivery Service: 1-800-HAWORTH. E-mail address: <docdelivery@haworthpress.com> Website: <http://www.HaworthPress.com> © 2006 by The Haworth Press, Inc. All rights reserved.]*

Laurie Grealish, RN, MN, Oncology Certificate, FRCNA, is Senior Lecturer in Nursing, University of Canberra, School of Health Sciences-Nursing, Canberra, ACT 2601, Australia.

[Haworth co-indexing entry note]: "Learning to Be a Professional: Two Models of Competence and Related Learning Strategies." Grealish, Laurie. Co-published simultaneously in *Journal of Religion, Spirituality & Aging* (The Haworth Pastoral Press, an imprint of The Haworth Press, Inc.) Vol. 18, No. 4, 2006, pp. 207-225; and: *Aging, Spirituality and Palliative Care* (ed: Elizabeth MacKinlay) The Haworth Pastoral Press, an imprint of The Haworth Press, Inc., 2006, pp. 207-225. Single or multiple copies of this article are available for a fee from The Haworth Document Delivery Service [1-800-HAWORTH, 9:00 a.m. - 5:00 p.m. (EST). E-mail address: docdelivery@haworthpress.com].

Available online at http://www.haworthpress.com/web/JRSA
doi:10.1300/J078v18n04_02

KEYWORDS. Competence, learning, practice, knowledge

INTRODUCTION

Professional education differs from education for the occupations by its delivery in the higher education (tertiary) sector. The academic focus of the tertiary sector has led to the privileging of propositional knowledge that is codified in the written word. Learning involves the application of theoretical understanding to practice experiences; apply theory to practice. In this approach, competence is a personal quality and requires acquisition of the requisite skills, knowledge, and attitude.

Review of the professional education literature reveals another approach, where practice is the focus for discovery and learning. This approach requires a broader view of competence, where competence is grounded in practice–it is operational. In the practice-based approach, knowledge that develops through practice experience is valued and learning occurs through analysis of the physical, emotional, and moral feelings, as they are experienced in practice. Rather than applying theory to practice, theory is used as a framework for analysing practice experiences.

BACKGROUND

Professional education has been based in the tertiary (university) sector on the grounds that professional practice requires the development of an expert knowledge base. Theory from the sciences and the arts, as well as theories that are unique to the professional discipline, are learned by students in readiness for the practice experience. Often, practice experiences are structured, with students being prepared to apply selected theories to the planned practice experience.

But practice settings are not ideal learning environments and they can run counter to those assumptions necessary to promote learning (Hughes, 1998). For example, many workplaces are structured to support hierarchical and authoritative approaches to work organization and practice rather than the egalitarian and cooperative approaches associated with learning (Hughes, 1998). In these models, the organization is more interested in the students' contribution to the work of the organization than their learning as a whole person. Service is prioritised over learning.

Contemporary health environments are concerned with staff short-ages (Davey, 2002; Edmond, 2001; Johnstone, 2002; Mitchell, 2003a), rising levels of mental distress in staff (Healy & McKay, 2000; John-stone, 2002), professional and personal struggle with ethical practice (Varcoe et al., 2004), and quality of service and service delivery (Glen, 1998). When health environments become learning environments, they present students with a world of conflicting and confusing values (Yong, 1996), create increased workloads and demands on staff (Freeth et al., 2001), and can engage students as defacto staff members rather than learners (Elliot, 2002a).

Students undertaking field experiences in the practice setting try to impress potential employers with their ability to do the work (Wilson, 1994). This may lead to attempts to hide inadequacies and avoidance of challenging situations where lack of ability may be apparent (Hughes, 1998).

The move to competency approaches to education have emerged from the apparent gap between what students learn in the classroom and what they need to know for work. The theory-practice gap plagues the nursing and allied health literature. Examples of the inadequacy of the-ory to adequately explain practice experiences are increasingly reach-ing the published literature. In one example, nurses working in cancer care struggle with the dual themes of intimacy and distance (Aranda, 2001). In this example, nurses learned through formal education that close nurse-patient relationships were to be avoided, making the imple-mentation of person-centred models of care more difficult.

The move to competence-based approaches to work in the health context is a response to the pressure of accountability (Alspach, 1992; Glen, 1998). The accountability systems emerge in response to percep-tions of expensive services, poor quality, or lack of alignment of service with community need (Eraut, 1998). In order to demonstrate account-ability for quality practice, some argue for the development of standards for performance measurement (Glen, 1998).

COMPETENCE

Competence is discussed in the literature as both potential to func-tion (personal) and actual performance (operational) (Alspach, 1992; Barnett, 1994; McAllister, 1998). The personal concept of competence is the potential to function that is based upon expert knowledge. Per-sonal competence is judged through examinations of theory using tests and essays. The operational concept of competence is grounded in practice. The actual performance is the basis for judgement. Operational competence provides a vehicle to demonstrate all aspects of practice, including caring (Cribb, 2001; Fosbinder, 1994).

The concept of competence continues to be problematic. The meanings (personal and operational) are used interchangeably (McAllister, 1998) and it is becoming clearer that competence is dependent upon the context of the situation (Arbon, 1995; Benner, 1982, 1984). There are suggestions that the concept of competence is both politically negotiated and socially situated (Eraut, 1998); the meaning of competence is constantly shifting.

In light of this ambiguity, there is growing dissatisfaction with the two conceptual models of competence. In the personal model, codified knowledge, or theory, is considered inadequate to explain clinical work; it excludes knowing related to caring practices (Cribb, 2001) whereas, in the operational model, a focus upon performance may lead to practice without thinking (Watson, 2002).

In addressing these shortcomings, Barnett (1994) suggests reflective knowing provides an epistemology that treats knowing seriously and skeptically, to embrace knowing while at the same time query it. Nurses in one study described this ability to be accurately aware of one's own expertise or limitations as insight (Pearson, Fitzgerald, & Walsh, 2002). This view accepts that all kinds of knowing can assist in understanding our world better, and recognizes that all forms of knowing are partial. It is consistent with those views emerging around continuing competence in nursing, where the principle of self-assessment is recommended as the basis for determining continued competence (Pearson et al., 1999). The notion of reflection, as described by Barnett (1994), continues to hold promise in the area of competence assessment (Chambers, 1998).

The ambiguous nature of the concept of competence is clearly revealed in the range of approaches currently available to assess competence. There appears to be general agreement that multiple approaches, within a continuous assessment framework, have usefulness (Chambers, 1998; Goding, 1997; Norman et al., 2002; Pearson, Fitzgerald, Walsh, & Borbasi, 2002; Redfern et al., 2002).

Most instruments currently available do not instil confidence in the students or practice assessors (Norman et al., 2002; Pearson, Fitzgerald, & Walsh, 2002). The instruments are difficult to apply and understand and there is little evidence that tests have been conducted to validate assessment instruments. The diversity of instruments available for the assessment of competence does not sit easily with national requirements (Norman et al., 2002). The challenge in assessing competence through a single instrument lies in the difficulty in operationalizing the concept (Chambers, 1998; Redfern et al., 2002; Sutton & Arbon, 1995; Watson et al., 2002). Some argue that a single definition of competence is important to advance assessment technology (Girot, 1993). However, in their research, Pearson et al. found that Australian nurses believed that no degree of valid inference about continuing competence is possible using a single indicator (Pearson, Fitzgerald, & Walsh, 2002).

There is a growing sentiment that levels of competence are illusory (Ashworth et al., 1999). Evidence is emerging to suggest that different levels of practice cannot be assessed using currently available instruments (Redfern et al., 2002). Lack of precise language, differences in use of language between groups, and the difficulty with verbal categorisations of actual practice phenomena can contribute to confusion around levels of attainment (Ashworth et al., 1999). There is consistent evidence of significant disagreement about 'essential' competencies between students and/or new graduates and preceptors, educators and managers (Canfield, 1982; Dolan, 2003; Marquis & Worth, 1992). The student and then, the new graduate are expected to negotiate these different expectations in order to 'survive' in the clinical arena.

LEARNING THROUGH PRACTICE

The value of health professions, such as nursing, is found in practice, rather than in a debate about theories derived from art and science (Bishop & Scudder, 1997). This view is reinforced by patients, who value clinical knowledge in the forms of experience and technical competence (Radwin, 2000). However, the contradictions between classroom (theory) and practice knowledge are rarely recognised in nursing curriculum (Clare, 1993).

Curriculum planners for education in the health professions are expected to provide some practical learning as part of the educational experience. The time in practice experience is usually short, with many assuming that practical knowledge will be easily 'picked up' on graduation (Edmond, 2001). But the workplace offers opportunities to learn knowledge that cannot be found in books. At the same time, the workplace cannot be controlled, leading to learning that is typically haphazard and unplanned (Boud & Walker, 1990). However, the designs for learning in the field are not as important as the experience it-self (Boud & Prosser, 2002).

Experience is broader than expertise (Arbon, 2004). Being experi-enced is a way of being, a positioning of one's self in practice or an out-look, and for experienced nurses, is connected to an understanding of who they are, what motivates them, and what they find fulfilling (Arbon, 2004). It is through experience, rather than classroom activi-ties, that critical thinking skill develops (Maynard, 1996). Theory about nursing, as lived by experienced nurses, derives its meanings and con-nections with a variety of situations–it is not stored in the mind in iso-lated and decontextualised form (Eraut, 1994).

The development of a learning culture in the workplace is seen as critical to effective learning (Egan & Abbott, 2002; Hart & Rotem, 1995). A clinical learning environment consists of variables that may contribute to a positive learning environment. Variables consider the extent to which:

- Staff are valued, acknowledged, and encouraged to take responsi-bility for their own practice (Hart & Rotem, 1995);
- Nurses enjoy their work and intend to pursue a career in nursing (Hart & Rotem, 1995);
- Staff understand and accept their role and responsibilities (Elliot, 2002a; Hart & Rotem, 1995; Mezirow, 1996);
- Clinical teacher and staff interaction facilitates or impedes im-proved practice (Hart & Rotem, 1995);
- Staff are friendly, caring, and supportive toward one another and students (Hart & Rotem, 1995; Papp et al., 2002);
- Clinical teacher and staff collaborate in teaching in the clinical set-ting (Davies et al., 1999; Freeth et al., 2001);
- Students are provided opportunities for learning (Hart & Rotem, 1995; Mezirow, 1996; Papp et al., 2002; Elliot, 2002);
- Students are aware of their influence on their learning environ-ment (Elliot, 2002b);
- The manager is supportive of learning (Dunn & Burnett, 1995);
- Students and staff are able to weigh evidence and arguments as ob-jectively as possible (Mezirow, 1996); and
- Students and staff are open to alternative perspectives (Mezirow, 1996).

Alert to learning through practice, students develop techniques in self-surveillance (Barnett, 1994; Glen, 1998). A form of normalizing judgement emerges, where a norm is established, against which individuals are measured, differentiated and judged (Gibson, 2001). Normalising judgement makes it possible to qualify, classify, measure, and compare the gaps between individuals to produce the concept of normal or good. Once this normalising process is put into motion, finer and finer differentiation and individuation occurs, objectifying and ranking practice/ people. Again, students want to be accepted by the work group and to be perceived as a good nurse and therefore work very hard to fit in (Chapman & Orb, 2001).

Although there are limitations to the various conceptual models, competence continues to be utilised in contemporary workplaces. Analysis of the teaching and learning practices required for two models of competence, personal and operational, provides insight into the ways that learning can be supported in the practice arena.

Personal Competence (Theory-Based Learning)

In this model, competence is about potential capability, based upon adequate academic achievements. The focus of learning is on theory, with the view that "theories provide the practitioner with a way to view client situations and thus serve as a vehicle for the interpretation and organization of information" (Raudonis & Acton, 1997, p. 138). Theory then directs the interpretation of relationships among the data and can guide practice decisions.

The assumptions about learning in this model, derived from the Scientific Measurement Model proposed by Hager and Butler (1996) and the Western Rational Tradition (Mezirow, 1996), include:

- Knowledge is certain, impersonal, context-free;
- Reality exists independently of linguistic representations of the world such as beliefs, experiences, statements, and theories;
- Truth is a matter of accuracy of representation;
- Logic and rationality are formal;
- Learning is focused on understanding disciplinary and subject perspectives;
- Problems are structured for the learner; and
- Theory is learned prior to practice.

Practical experiences are usually arranged so that recently learned theory can be applied. Students attend field placements with the support of a clinical teacher, appointed by the university.

Personal competence is separated into three parts to facilitate teaching. Cognitive, psychomotor, and affective aspects of competence are developed separately, with the expectation that they will come together in the practice arena. Cognitive aspects of competence are developed through classroom learning. Psychomotor or technical skills are selected based on clinical work (Kieffer, 1984) and broken down into parts for learning in the laboratory setting and assessment in the workplace (Johnson et al., 2001). Affective aspects are developed through study of moral and ethical theories, and through classroom discussion. Critical thinking skills are learned in the context of argument development and evaluation.

In this framework, finding the best way to provide care is the goal. Evidence-based practice and quality improvement approaches are highly valued. However, in health, the theory-based framework is dominated by the positivist, biomedical paradigm (Cribb, 2001). Best is presented in the form of propositional knowledge, produced through research methods that satisfy the methodological rigours of positivism, which include control, measurement, categorisation, and prediction. The risk with the best way approach is that other forms of knowledge, such as tacit, personal, and practical, that are produced through other methods, may be rendered invisible or excluded (Mitchell & Pilkington, 1999). This means that the human and ethical aspects of practice require focused consideration when evaluating professional actions in the personal model of competence to ensure usefulness (Mitchell, 1997).

In this model, students are responsible to realize the potential of the learning experience. They bring intent, or personal determination, which provides a particular orientation within a given situation (Boud & Walker, 1990). Intent can act as a filter or magnifier; it offers a frame of reference from which an experience is viewed, influencing what the learner notices and what they do in response (Boud & Walker, 1990). The clinical teacher helps learners clarify their intent, and identify learning opportunities appropriate to their intent.

Clinical teachers are usually recognized expert clinicians, employed by the university, to teach the students in the field. Academics, in general, are removed from the clinical encounter. Here, the instructional paradigm is privileged (Fear et al., 2003). The teacher, in collaboration with the student, establishes deliberate learning objectives in the practice setting. However, there is a risk that the range of teachable moments that emerge in the clinical experience may be overlooked in the rush to structure learning to fit with pre-existing objectives (Morton-Cooper & Palmer, 1993).

The clinicians, who also have an educative role, share their practice with students through explanation. This type of teaching can be time consuming (Wotton & Gonda, 2004) and, as such, creates tensions between service and learning work. Students learn the way that practice is done in that workplace, with responses to their questions focused on explaining why things are done in a particular way. Rather than challenging practice, by suggesting other ways, students uncritically adopt the paradigm view of the workplace (Plsek, 1997), learning to fit in. There is evidence that students learn very quickly how to play the game known as 'don't rock the boat' by becoming what or who the clinical teacher and staff wanted them to be (Chapman & Orb, 2001).

Students learning in the clinical practice setting quickly learn that the knowledge gained in the classroom is not adequate to explain their practice experiences (Clare, 1993). There is an acceptance, almost an expectation, that practice is different to theory and students, trying to fit in, generally do not challenge the differences that they encounter (Grealish & Trevitt, 2005). An important teaching strategy to bridge the practice-theory gap in these situations is reflection (Hart, 1997). The processes for reflection are described in Table 1.

Reflection enables correction of distortions in beliefs and errors in problem solving (Mezirow, 1990). Learning the skills of reflection can provide students with a life-long learning strategy for continued analysis and learning about practice (Morton-Cooper & Palmer, 1993).

TABLE 1. Reflection

In individual reflection, after the incident, the following guide may be used.

RETURN TO THE EXPERIENCE. Over the course of a day, many experiences have occurred. Chose one experience for analysis based upon feeling stymied or puzzled by the event. Recall specific detail of what happened, including who was involved.

IDENTIFICATION OF PERSONAL FEELINGS that occurred in response to the practice incident. Conflicting feelings that changed over time are notable.

SEARCHING FOR MEANING in the event requires using feelings experienced as a trigger to analyze the personal response to the incident. Consider what happened in light of what was expected to happen.

VALIDATION. The meanings that develop following analysis of the event are then validated. Validation can take the form of verifying meaning with involved individuals. It can also occur by evaluating personal understanding of the event in light of current literature.

LEARNING. How this reflection has assisted learning is revealed in the outcome—how will practice change in light of this new knowledge?

Finally, time in the practice setting is usually limited, and in such circumstances, students generally aim to experience as many different situations as possible. In doing so, they do not develop learning sets. Learning sets are the repeated responses of the professional that inform the development of the habitual skilled body (Edmond, 2001; Benner & Wrubel, 1989). The development of the habitual skilled body is expected to occur once the student graduates and is working as a professional.

Operational Competence (Practice-Based Learning)

Operational competence is not separated into parts to facilitate learning and assessment. In the operational view of competence, it is accepted that the separation of competence into cognitive, affective, and psychomotor domains for assessment may not give a true indication of competence (Alspach, 1992). All three aspects of competence can be learned at once through analysis of practice. Theory acts as a guide to think about or analyze, rather than control, practice; it is considered tentative and open to change (Barnett, 1994; Carper, 1978; Fujimura, 1996). Theory, including personal beliefs and values, influences practice and in turn, practice influences theory (Cody & Mitchell, 1992; Eraut, 1994).

In thinking about operational competence and practice-based learning, the learning paradigm emerges as different to the instructional paradigm (Fear et al., 2003). The learning paradigm is focused on deep learning as personal engagement in experience. Learning is inherent in human nature and not considered a special activity (Wenger, 1998). Learning is influenced by the socio-emotional context in which it occurs (Boud, 1993, cited in Boud & Prosser, 2002), therefore attention to the environment and personal feelings are important aspects of learning.

The assumptions about learning within the operational competence model are that learning:

- Is shaped by the frame of reference that delimits perception, cognition, and feelings by predisposing our intentions, expectations, and purposes (Mezirow, 1996);
- Is the process of using past interpretations to negotiate a new or a revised interpretation of the meaning of one's experience (Mezirow, 1996; Wenger, 1998);
- Is a matter of social energy and power, thriving on identification and dependent on negotiability (Wenger, 1998);

- Is a matter of imagination, dependent on processes of orientation, reflection, and exploration to place our identities and practices in a broader context (Mezirow, 1996; Wenger, 1998);
- Involves the whole person in a dynamic interplay of participation and reification (Wenger, 1998);
- Is relational, always situated in a context (Boud & Prosser, 2002); and
- Involves our own experience of participation and reification as well as forms of competence defined by our communities (Wenger, 1998).

Students work as part of the health care team and practical learning occurs through work experience. As identified by Hughes (1998), there is a risk that work can overtake learning in this model. Further, there is a risk that, when only clinical staff facilitate learning, there will be an uncritical passing down of thought systems from one generation to the next (Eraut, 1994; Plsek, 1997). The key appears to be establishing a learning environment that provides the intellectual freedom to challenge practice assumptions.

People, including students, are meaning-makers (Butler, 1996; Fear, 2003; Goding, 1997). They create personal meaning from their experiences. Evidence is collected to fit with closely held frames of reference or known concepts. The goal for learning is discovery; the learning process is emancipatory in nature. Social constraints, such as conceptual approaches and theories, are illuminated for critique and possible change (Clare, 2003). Openness to alternative perspectives provides opportunity to "both transcend the power structures embedded in knowledge frameworks and create anew the situations before us" (Barnett, 1994, p. 180). By establishing practice experiences as cases for analysis, understanding can be enhanced and opportunities for change become possible (Bishop & Scudder, 1997). In this approach, those practices deemed as best are also open to analysis (Smith & Sutton, 1999).

Critical thinking skills are essential in this approach. This is consistent with most theory about higher education (Barnett, 1994; Glen, 1995; Harden, 1996; Kim, 1999; Meerbeau, 1992; Schank, 1990; Smith, 2001). As with personal competence, skills in reflection (Bechtel, Davidhizer, & Bradshaw, 1999; Boud, Keogh, & Walker, 1985; Fernandez, 1997; Hart 1997; Milligan, 1998), where all forms of knowledge required for practice (tacit, propositional, practical, and experimental) can be examined, are crucial.

Critical reflection (Freeth et al., 2001; Mezirow, 1990; Mitchell, 1995), where knowledge from various paradigms provides the frameworks to analyze practice, is also necessary for learning from practice. Unlike reflection, critical reflection is not done alone. Examining practices through analysis requires intellectual effort and encouragement from peers (Eraut, 1994). Dialogue and argument are essential components to learning through analysis (Barnett, 1994). Through such discussion, the holistic, relational, and problematic nature of learning is revealed (Boud & Prosser, 2002) and frameworks for understanding can be developed.

Challenging practice assumptions, through critical reflection, requires development of the process of seeing the difference and of integrating the unfamiliar with the familiar (Mitchell, 2003b). A clinical guide, preferably not a member of the health organization, could assist in developing these processes (Andrews & Roberts, 2003). By identifying multiple perspectives, or paradigms, for analysis of practice experience, the clinical guide can help students (and staff) to see the inconsistencies that may exist in current practice regimes (Barnett, 1994). Mascord (1988) does this with great effect in the article about Mrs. Baird, who received care from five different nurses, practising from five different nursing frameworks, over five days. The ways that the conceptual models of nursing could influence nursing care, with remarkable differences, is revealed to readers as they follow Mrs. Baird's journey over the week.

The outsider, academic nurse, could support student learning, and provide an encouraging environment in several ways:

- Work closely with the clinical leader/manager to determine shared aims and expected outcomes for students and clinical staff following student experience;
- Discuss, with staff, the principles underpinning learning and how these may be different to other models;
- Encourage group discussion of practice by students and staff;
- Take interest in the practice issues raised by staff; and
- Encourage critical thinking about those issues.

A suggested guide for critical reflection in groups is provided in Table 2.

Another strategy that challenges practice assumptions is to move from one learning community to another. For example, when student nurses moved from hospital to community settings, the experience resulted in broader perspectives of health and illness, enhanced assessment and interpersonal skills, and an increased awareness of the nature

TABLE 2. Critical Reflection

During group discussion, the following guide may be used:

- Students and staff describe practice incidents as fully as possible in a 'story telling' style (shared stories and experiences are encouraged).
- The individual sharing the story identifies why the incident was important or remembered over other incidents.
- The group, as well as the individual, discusses the significant aspects, and how these were interpreted, as it evolved in the incident.
- The group then discusses the impact of the significant aspects, and how these were interpreted, as it evolved in the incident.
- The outsider, in collaboration with the group, compares the nurses' intentions and actual practice–through this exercise distortions, inconsistencies, and incongruence between values/beliefs and practice, intentions and actions, and clients' needs and nurses' actions can be revealed for further consideration.
- The outsider then asks the group to consider how the situation might be different if another theory was used to understand the event/incident.

of the relationship between the consumer and provider of care (Conger et al., 1999).

One benefit of the operational competence model is that, through their presence in the clinical field, academics stay in touch with practice matters, important for research work (Downie et al., 2001). Through collaborative learning activities, scholarship in practice develops (Davies et al., 1999; Downie et al., 2001). From this work, new practice frameworks, that more effectively address consumer concerns and health, rather than treatment approaches, can emerge (Corner, 1997). When work practices are reconsidered in light of new paradigms, shared models of continuous practice development can grow (Parsons & Mott, 2003; Ward & McCormack, 2000). Creativity, as a competence, is valued (Glen, 1998).

DISCUSSION

Personal competence is the dominant model in contemporary tertiary education and derives from a long tradition of valuing expert knowledge. It has value in that theory can guide practice and reflection. Reflection is an accepted learning strategy that has emerged from the personal competence approach.

However the limitations of theory-based learning continue to disappoint students. Theories provide, at best, incomplete explanations of practice, leaving students vulnerable at the time that they need most support (Eraut, 1994). The focus on theory, and classroom activities, leads to decreased time in the practice setting and students often delay the development of the habitual skilled body until the first few years of their practice careers. Finally, the acceptance of theory as fact, which commonly occurs in undergraduate education, has the potential to inhibit creative development of practice in the workplace.

Operational competence has been avoided in professional education. A primary reason for this is the risk of 'occupational vocationalism' (Glen, 1995). The operational competence model, applied without critical reflection, can reduce education to training (Milligan, 1998; Watson, 2002). However, the practice of teaching theory as fact within education and using theory to drive curricula removes the tentative and guiding contribution that a theory can make to a profession (Morse, 1995).

There is a need for approaches to teaching and learning that provide graduates with conceptual frameworks that guide practice, and foster opportunities for discovery of occupationally relevant concepts that are embedded within practice work. Practice-based learning, associated with the model of operational competence offers opportunities for practice communities to analyze their practice using critical reflection. With the addition of academic presence, there is potential support and facilitated critique of practice from a range of perspectives and theories.

CONCLUSION

Students learn differently when the focus is on understanding or performance (Mezirow, 1990). Due to the vocational character of operational competence, there is a perception within academia that this approach devalues the academic contribution to learning. Privileging propositional knowledge over other forms of knowledge serves to continue to keep theory and practice separate. The learning strategies associated with operational competence, reflection, critical reflection, and the development of learning sets, provide opportunity to support students on their journey to becoming a health professional.

REFERENCES

Alspach, G. (1992). Concern and confusion over competence. *Critical Care Nurse, 12, 4*, 9-11.

Andrews, M., & Roberts, D. (2003). Supporting student nurses learning in and through clinical practice: The role of clinical guide. *Nurse Education Today, 23*, 474-481.

Aranda, S. (2001). Silent voices, hidden practices: Exploring undiscovered aspects of cancer nursing. *International Journal of Palliative Care, 7, 4*, 178-185.

Arbon, P. (1995). Nursing exemplars: Are they de-contextualised? *Nursing Inquiry, 2,* 185-6

Arbon, P. (2004). Understanding experience in nursing. *Journal of Clinical Nursing, 13,* 150-157.

Ashworth, P., Gerrish, K., Hargreaves, J., & McManus, M. (1999). 'Levels' of attainment in nursing practice: Reality or illusion? *Journal of Advanced Nursing, 30, 1,* 159-168.

Barnett, R. (1994). *The limits of competence: Knowledge, higher education, and society.* Buckingham: SRHE & Open University Press.

Bechtel, G. A., Davidhizer, R., & Bradshaw, M. J. (1999). Problem-based learning in a competency-based world. *Nurse Education Today, 19*, 182-187.

Benner, P. (1982). Issues in competency-based testing. *Nursing Outlook, 30*, 303-309.

Benner, P. (1984). From novice to expert: Excellence and power in clinical nursing practice. Menlo Park: Addison-Wesley.

Benner, P., & Wrubel, J. (1989). The primacy of caring: Stress and coping in health and illness. Menlo Park: Addison-Wesley.

Bishop, A. H., & Scudder, J. (1997). Nursing as a practice rather than an art or science. *Nursing Outlook, 45, 2*, 82-85.

Boud, D., Keogh, R., & Walker, D. (1985). Promoting reflection in learning: A model. In Boud, D., Keogh, R., & Walker, D. (Eds.). *Reflection: Turning experience into learning.* New York: Kogan Page.

Boud, D., & Prosser, M. (2002). Appraising new technologies for learning: A framework for development. *Education Media International, 39, 3/4*, 237-245.

Boud, D., & Walker, D. (1990). Making the most of experience. *Studies in Continuing Education, 12, 2*, 61-80.

Butler, J. (1996). Professional development: Practice as text, reflection as process, and self as locus. *Australian Journal of Education, 40, 3*, 265-283.

Canfield, A. (1982). Controversy over clinical competencies. *Heart & Lung, 11, 3,* 197-199.

Carper, B. A. (1978). Fundamental patterns of knowing in nursing. *Advances in Nursing Science, 1, 1*, 13-23.

Chambers, A. (1998). Some issues in the assessment of clinical practice: A review of the literature. *Journal of Clinical Nursing, 7, 3*, 201-208.

Chapman, R., & Orb, A. (2001). Coping strategies in clinical practice: The nursing students' lived experience. *Contemporary Nurse, 11*, 95-102.

Clare, J. (1993). Change the curriculum—Or transform the conditions of practice? *Nurse Education Today, 13*, 282-286.

Clare, J. (2003). Writing critical research. In Clare, J., & Hamilton, H. (Eds.). *Writing research: Transforming data into text.* Sydney: Churchill Livingstone.

Cody, W. K., & Mitchell, G. J. (1992). Parse's theory as a model for practice: The cutting edge. *Advances in Nursing Science, 15, 2,* 52-65.

Conger, C. O., Baldwin, J. H., Abegglen, J., & Callister, L. (1999). The shifting sands of health care delivery: Curriculum revision and integration of community health nursing. *Journal of Nursing Education, 38, 7,* 304-311.

Corner, J. (1997). Beyond survival rates and side effects: Cancer nursing as therapy. *Cancer Nursing, 20, 1,* 3-11.

Cribb, A. (2001). Knowledge and caring: A philosophical and personal perspective. In Corner, J., Bailey, C. (Eds.). *Cancer nursing: Care in context.* Oxford: Blackwell Science.

Davey, L. (2002). Nurses eating nurses: The caring profession which fails to nurture its own. *Contemporary Nurse, 13, 2-3,* 192-197.

Davies, C., Welham, V., Glover, A., Jones, L., & Murphy, F. (1999). Teaching in practice. *Nursing Standard, 13, 35,* 33-38.

Dolan, G. (2003). Assessing student competence: Will we ever get it right? *Journal of Clinical Nursing, 12, 1,* 132-141.

Downie, J., Orb, A., Wyndaden, D., McGowan, S., Seeman, Z., & Olgivie, S. (2001). A practice-research model for collaborative partnership. *Collegian, 8, 4,* 27-32.

Dunn. S., & Burnett, P. (1995). The development of a clinical learning environment scale. *Journal of Advanced Nursing, 22,* 1166-1173.

Edmond, C. (2001). A new paradigm for practice education. *Nurse Education Today, 21,* 251-259.

Egan, K. A., & Abbott, P. (2002). Interdisciplinary team training: Preparing new employees for the specialty of hospice and palliative care. *Journal of Hospice & Palliative Care Nursing, 4, 3,* 161-171.

Elliot, M. (2002a). The clinical environment: A source of stress for undergraduate nurses. *Australian Journal of Advanced Nursing, 20, 1,* 34-38.

Elliot, M. (2002b). Clinical education: A challenging component of undergraduate nursing education. *Contemporary Nurse, 12, 1,* 69-77.

Eraut, M. (1994). *Developing professional knowledge and competence.* London: The Falmer Press.

Eraut, M. (1998). Concepts of competence. *Journal of Interprofessional Care, 12, 2,* 127-139.

Fear, F., Doberneck, D., Robinson, C., Fear, K., & Barr, R. (2003). Meaning making and "The Learning Paradigm": A provocative idea in practice. *Innovative Higher Education, 27, 3,* 151-168.

Fernandez, E. (1997). Just 'doing the observations': Reflective practice in nursing. *British Journal of Nursing, 6, 16,* 939-943.

Fosbinder, D. (1994). Patient perceptions of nursing care: An emerging theory of interpersonal competence. *Journal of Advanced Nursing, 20,* 1085-1093.

Freeth, D., Reeves, S., Goreham, C., Parker, P., Haynes, S., & Pearson, S. (2001). 'Real life' clinical learning on an interprofessional training ward. *Nurse Education Today, 21,* 366-372.

Fujimura, J. (1996). *Crafting science: A sociohistory of the quest for the genetics of cancer.* Harvard University Press: Cambridge, MA.

Gibson, T. (2001). Nurses and medication error: A discursive reading of the literature. *Nursing Inquiry, 8, 2,* 108-117.

Girot, E. (1993). Assessment of competence in clinical practice: A phenomenological approach. *Journal of Advanced Nursing, 18*, 114-119.

Glen, S. (1995). Towards a new model of nursing education. *Nurse Education Today, 15*, 90-95.

Glen, S. (1998). Emotional and motivational tendencies: The key to quality nursing care? *Nursing Ethics, 5, 1*, 36-42.

Goding, L. (1997). Can degree level practice be assessed? *Nurse Education Today, 17*, 158-161.

Grealish, L., & Trevitt, C. (2005). Developing a professional identity: Student nurses in the workplace. *Contemporary Nurse, 1-2*, 137-150.

Hager, P., & Butler, J. (1996). Two models of educational assessment. *Assessment & Evaluation in Higher Education, 21, 4*, 367-378.

Harden, J. (1996). Enlightenment, empowerment, and emancipation: The case for critical pedagogy in nurse education. *Nurse Education Today, 16*, 32-37.

Hart, G. (1997). Clinical teaching strategies to encourage reflective practice. *International Journal of PEPE Inc, 1, 1*, 53-67.

Hart, G., & Rotem, A. (1995). The clinical learning environment: Nurses' perceptions of professional development in clinical settings. *Nurse Education Today, 15*, 3-10.

Healy, C. M., & McKay, M. F. (2000). Nursing stress: The effects of coping strategies and job satisfaction in a sample of Australian nurses. *Journal of Advanced Nursing, 31, 3*, 681-688.

Hughes, C. (1998). Practicum learning: Perils of the authentic workplace. *Higher Education Research and Development, 17, 2*, 207-227.

Johnson, M., Marden, J., Day, E., & Chang, S. (2001). Nursing skill assessment within populations: Scale development and testing. *Contemporary Nurse, 10, 1-2*, 46-57.

Johnstone, M. (2002). Poor working conditions and the capacity of nurses to provide moral care. *Contemporary Nurse, 12*, 7-15.

Kieffer, J. S. (1984). Selecting technical skills to teach for competency. *Journal of Nursing Education, 23, 5*, 198-203.

Kim, H. (1999). Critical reflective inquiry for knowledge development in nursing practice. *Journal of Advanced Nursing, 29, 5*, 1205-1212.

Marquis, B., & Worth, C. (1992). The relationship among multiple assessments of nursing education outcomes. *Journal of Nursing Education, 31, 1*, 33-38.

Mascord, P. (1988). Five days: Five nursing theories. *Australian Journal of Advanced Nursing, 6, 2*, 13-15.

Maynard, C. A. (1996). Relationship of critical thinking ability to professional nurse competence. *Journal of Nursing Education, 35, 1*, 12-18.

McAllister, M. (1998). Competency standards: Clarifying the issues. *Contemporary Nurse, 7, 3, 131-137.*

Meerabeau, L. (1992). Tacit nursing knowledge: An untapped resource or a methodological headache? *Journal of Advanced Nursing, 17*, 108-112.

Mezirow, J. (1990). How critical reflection triggers transformative learning. In Mezirow, J. (Ed.). *Fostering critical reflection in adulthood: A guide to transformative and emancipatory learning.* San Francisco: Jossey-Bass.

Mezirow, J. (1996). Contemporary paradigms of learning. *Adult Education Quarterly, 46(3)*, 158-173.

Milligan, F. (1998). Defining and assessing competence: The distraction of outcomes and the importance of educational process. *Nurse Education Today*, *18*, 273-280.

Mitchell, G. J. (1995). Reflection: The key to breaking with tradition. *Nursing Science Quarterly*, *8*, *2*, 57-58.

Mitchell, G. J. (1997). Questioning evidence-based practice for nursing. *Nursing Science Quarterly*, *19*, *4*, 154-155.

Mitchell, G. J. (2003a). Nursing shortage or nursing famine: Looking beyond the numbers? *Nursing Science Quarterly*, *16*, *3*, 219-224.

Mitchell, G. J. (2003b). Abstractions and particulars: Learning theory for practice. *Nursing Science Quarterly*, *16*, *4*, 310-314.

Mitchell, G. J., & Pilkington, F. B. (1999). A dialogue on the comparability of research paradigms–And other theoretical things. *Nursing Science Quarterly*, *12*, *4*, 283-289.

Morse, J. M. (1995). Nursing scholarship: Sense and sensibility. *Nursing Inquiry*, *3*, 74-82.

Morton-Cooper, A., & Palmer, A. (1993). *Mentoring and preceptorship: A guide to support roles in clinical practice.* Oxford: Blackwell Science.

Norman, I., Watson, R., Murrells, T., Calman, L., & Redfern, S. (2002). The validity and reliability of methods to assess the competence to practise of pre-registration nursing and midwifery students. *International Journal of Nursing Studies*, *39*, 133-145.

Papp, I., Markkanen, M., & von Bonsdorff, M. (2002). Clinical environment as a learning environment: Student nurses' perceptions concerning clinical learning experiences. *Nurse Education Today*, *23*, 262-268.

Parsons, M., & Mott, S. (2003). Royal Rehabilitation Centre Sydney: Towards Clinical Development Units (Nursing). *Collegian*, *10*, *1*, 27-29

Pearson, A., Fitzgerald, M., Borbasi, S., Walsh, K., Parkes, R., Lazarevic, L., & Mather, G. (1999). *A study to identify the indicators of continuing competence in nursing: Final report.* Canberra: ANCI.

Pearson, A., Fitzgerald, M., Walsh, K., & Borbasi, S. (2002). Continuing competence and the regulation of nursing practice. *Journal of Nursing Management*, *10*, *6*, 357-363.

Pearson, A., Fitzgerald, M., & Walsh, K. (2002). Nurses' views on competency indicators for Australian nursing. *Collegian*, *9*, *1*, 36-40.

Plsek, P. E. (1997). Collaborating across organizational boundaries to improve the quality of care. *American Journal of Infection Control*, *25*, 85-95.

Radwin, L. (2000). Oncology patients' perceptions of quality nursing care. *Research in Nursing & Health*, *23*, 179-190.

Raudonis, B., & Acton, G. (1997). Theory-based nursing practice. *Journal of Advanced Nursing*, *26*, 138-145.

Redfern, S., Norman, I., Calman, L., Watson, R., & Murrells, T. (2002). Assessing competence to practice in nursing: A review of the literature. *Research Papers in Education 17*, *1*, 51-77.

Schank, M. J. (1990). Wanted: Nurses with critical thinking skills. *The Journal of Continuing Education in Nursing*, *21*, *2*, 86-89.

Smith, A. (2001). Nursing in a time of change: A case for critical thinking. *Contemporary Nurse*, *10*, 194-200.

Smith, C., & Sutton, F. (1999). Best practice: What it is and what it is not. *International Journal of Nursing Practice*, *5*, 100-105.

Sutton, F., & Arbon, P. (1995). Australian nursing–Moving forward? Competencies and the nursing profession. *Nurse Education Today, 14*, 388-393.

Varcoe, C., Doane, G., Pauly, B., Rodney, P., Storch, J. L., Mahoney, K., McPherson, G., Brown, H., & Starzomski, R. (2004). Ethical practice in nursing: Working the in-between. *Journal of Advanced Nursing, 45, 3*, 316-325.

Ward, C., & McCormack, B. (2000). Creating an adult learning culture through practice development. *Nurse Education Today, 20*, 259-266.

Watson, R. (2002). Clinical competence: Starship Enterprise or straitjacket? *Nurse Education Today, 22*, 476-480.

Watson, R., Stimpson, A., Topping, A., & Porock, D. (2002). Clinical competence assessment in nursing: A systematic review of the literature. *Journal of Advanced Nursing, 39, 5*, 421-431.

Wenger, E. (1998). *Communities of practice: Learning, meaning, and identity*. Cambridge: Cambridge University Press.

Wilson, M. E. (1994). Nursing student perspective of learning in a clinical setting. *Journal of Nursing Education, 33, 2*, 81-86.

Wooton, K., & Gonda, J. (2004). Clinician and student evaluation of a collaborative clinical teaching model. *Nurse Education in Practice, 4*, 120-127.

Yong, V. (1996). 'Doing clinical': The lived experience of nursing students. *Contemporary Nurse, 5*, 73-79.

"Till Death Us Do Part":
Issues of Fidelity in End of Life Care

Margaret O'Connor, RN, DN, MN, BTheol
Susan Lee, RN, MBioeth, BAppSciAdvNurs (Edu),
DipAppSci (Nurs)

SUMMARY. This paper was born of the experience of caring for a loved one at the end of life. The sense of being torn between accepting one's lot and wishing for something "other" is at the heart of the concept described as "intimate fidelity." Intimate fidelity is discussed as part of a multi-layered concept of fidelity, embracing aspects of the professional caring relationship, and which builds into a value that shapes the fabric of the community.

Academic literature fails to address this understanding of fidelity, so with some creativity, we turned to popular literature–novels and biographies–to find rich understandings of the concept of fidelity. Then following a traditional system of thematic analysis, three aspects of the

---

Margaret O'Connor, RN, DN, MN, BTheol, is Vivian Bullwinkel Chair in Nursing, Palliative Care, School of Nursing and Midwifery, Monash University, P.O. Box 527, Frankston 3199, Australia (E-mail: Margaret.OConnor@med.monash.edu.au).

Susan Lee, RN, MBioeth, BAppSci AdvNurs. (Edu), DipAppSci (Nurs), is Senior Lecturer, School of Nursing and Midwifery, Monash University, P.O. Box 527, Frankston 3199, Australia (E-mail: Susan.Lee@med.monash.edu.au).

[Haworth co-indexing entry note]: " 'Till Death Us Do Part': Issues of Fidelity in End of Life Care." O'Connor, Margaret, and Susan Lee. Co-published simultaneously in *Journal of Religion, Spirituality & Aging* (The Haworth Pastoral Press, an imprint of The Haworth Press, Inc.) Vol. 18, No. 4, 2006, pp. 227-245; and: *Aging, Spirituality and Palliative Care* (ed: Elizabeth MacKinlay) The Haworth Pastoral Press, an imprint of The Haworth Press, Inc., 2006, pp. 227-245. Single or multiple copies of this article are available for a fee from The Haworth Document Delivery Service [1-800-HAWORTH, 9:00 a.m. - 5:00 p.m. (EST). E-mail address: docdelivery@haworthpress.com].

Available online at http://www.haworthpress.com/web/JRSA
doi:10.1300/J078v18n04_03

concept of fidelity are presented, in the context of caring for loved ones, professional caring, and caring in the community. *[Article copies available for a fee from The Haworth Document Delivery Service: 1-800-HAWORTH. E-mail address: <docdelivery@haworthpress.com> Website: <http://www.HaworthPress. com> © 2006 by The Haworth Press, Inc. All rights reserved.]*

KEYWORDS. Fidelity, caring, end of life, community

INTRODUCTION

This paper was born out of extensive reflection on the lengthy experience of caring for an elderly aunt by one of the authors. Being brought face to face with the "duty" to visit, to stand with her and witness the state of her pain, frustrated by my powerlessness to soothe her, desiring for this duty to be over, but needing to see it through; sensing that this fidelity was somehow her lifeline. Even though the author's debt to her was immense from an earlier time . . . she felt she received *nothing* from this relationship during this time . . . and she vividly recalls an almost physical sense of dragging herself to frequently visit her.

This experience of being torn between accepting one's lot as a consequence of a relationship, and wishing for something "other" is at the heart of the concept described as "intimate fidelity"–that caring response that emerges from within an existing relationship. Intimate fidelity does not stand alone as an individual experience however, but can be viewed as part of a multi-layered concept of fidelity and perhaps a developing model, that embraces aspects of the professional caring relationship, and which builds into a value that shapes the fabric of the community (Figure 1).

PHILOSOPHICAL, MORAL, AND LITERATURE FOUNDATIONS OF A CONCEPT OF FIDELITY

An initial literature search on the word fidelity related it to the commitment made by the partners in a marriage/commitment ceremony. This idealistic understanding of the concept is set in the positive and hope-filled emotion of this ritual in the lives of the people concerned. Even though there is other literature describing caring roles and the bur-

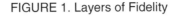

FIGURE 1. Layers of Fidelity

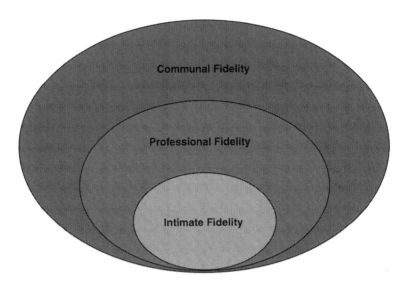

dens and benefits of caring there is no academic literature that addresses the living out of the promise of fidelity–that of the (often) other end of the relationship, where the balance of the partnership has changed and one partner is required to support the other in different ways. It has taken some creativity to pull out some foundational understandings of the word "fidelity" across a diverse range of literature.

In *mythological writings*, in particular the legend of King Arthur, fidelity was used in relation to conjugal faithfulness in the description of a ladies cloak, given to the king to test the fidelity of his wife. On a faithful wife, the fidelity mantle would look beautiful; however, on those disloyal to their husbands, as the faithless Queen Guinevere found, its colour would change to black and it would appear in tatters (Brewer, 1898).

At a broad level, in *biological sciences*, the term fidelity describes the constancy that exists in nature in the accurate copying of genetic material when cells divide. At a cellular level, the copied cell looks and functions exactly like its parent. Furthermore, in the *physical sciences*, when an electronic system such as an amplifier faithfully reproduces sound outputs that have the same desired characteristics as its sound input, it is known as a 'hi fidelity' system (Delbridge, 1986).

Professionally, in *bio-ethics*, fidelity is used to describe the observance of promises and loyalty from the perspective of duty, character, and caring. Beauchamp and Childress (1989) discuss fidelity as a rule of relationships, particularly those between physicians and their patients, where there is at least an implied promise that the physician will "seek the patient's welfare" (Beauchamp & Childress, 1989, p. 342). Pellegrino and Thomasma (1993) also place fidelity centrally in the maintenance of relationships, particularly to the character of health care professionals and how they approach trust in relationships with patients.

In contrast to these authors, Ramsey argues that fidelity is a central moral principle based on a *religious notion* of promises being a covenant "with the meaning it gives to righteousness between man and man" (Ramsey, 1970, p. xii). Ramsey places his discussion of loyalty and faithfulness in the context of medical relationships as a covenant not just between people, but also with God, and would in the same way view the care of the dying by family members. Of them he declares that the bonds of love and filial duty strengthen the covenant, and the promise to care, that binds their relationship.

Thus, many complex understandings of fidelity were found, not many of them helpful in explicating the concept as experienced in a caring relationship when a person is dying. In the end, we turned to popular literature–novels and biographies–those that document the experience of another; books that one devours late into the night to suck the marrow of the author's experience in an attempt to affirm/confirm one's own. That literature is rich indeed in understandings of fidelity.

Storytelling is a basic element in human life–reading the papers, telling the tales of the day to a family member, even television soaps all provide the vehicle for retrospective reflection on the experience to find meaning, and to foretell future actions (Borkan et al., 1999). Storytelling performs a communal role in being a vehicle of care for another, because sharing the stories can be cathartic for both the storyteller and the listener and contain the potential to change behaviour. Arthur Franks (1995) also describes the use of narrative in learning models of medical education–"to increase the potency of our care for patients, to allow our personal experiences to strengthen the empathic bond with those who suffer" (p. xii). Stories of suffering, in particular, bring us beyond our own world, and give the capacity to step into another's shoes to employ "sympathetic imagination" (Kearney, 2002). It is this literature that formed the basis of understanding intimate fidelity that will now be pursued in this paper. Comment will also be provided on aspects of professional fidelity and fidelity as it should be understood within a communal framework (see Figure 1).

The books reviewed contained a mix of genre, but mostly that of a testimony, written by the carer, some diarised, some written in retrospect. One of the books is a novel, though one wonders how it could have been written without intimate knowledge of the scenario depicted. A range of relationships was chosen, to add contrast, but also to illustrate that fidelity is a concept not unique to a marital relationship. Many books could have been chosen, but five have been used here that highlighted the concept of fidelity, and are stories that have touched the authors, personally and professionally and were:

- Orchard, Sonia (2003). *Something more wonderful: A true story.* Hodder, Sydney. A young woman's experience of the journey to death of her 31-year-old friend Emma (and mother of a two-year-old child) with liver cancer;
- Bayley, John (1998). *Iris: A memoir of Iris Murdoch.* Abacus books, London. John's experiences of caring for Iris Murdoch, his wife of more than 40 years, as she sank into Alzheimer's disease.
- Cracknell, Ruth (2000). *Journey from Venice: A memoir.* Penguin Books, Melbourne. Journaling the horrendous last months of life for her husband Eric, again of 40 years, suddenly diagnosed with cancer while traveling.
- Jennings, Kate (2003). *Moral hazard.* Picador, Sydney. A story about this young wife whose husband Bailey is much older and the balancing of his increasing need because of advancing Alzheimer's and her own working life.
- De Beauvoir, Simone (1964). *A very easy death.* Penguin Books, London. The account of this famous philosopher's care for her mother in her final days.

Following a traditional system of thematic analysis which may include highlighting key words and phrases, looking for emphases and themes within and between texts, three aspects of the concept of fidelity emerged. There are possibly many more, but from the chosen literature, these are what emerged:

- Immersion–"life on hold"
- Commitment–"a new depth"
- Persistence–"seeing things through"

ANALYSIS

Immersion–"Life on Hold"

The theme of 'immersion' describes the way that the carers in these stories became deeply involved in their unsought new role of caring, experiencing the loss of the old relationship and the meaninglessness of time. Each of the stories graphically describes the time when the relationship altered: a diagnosis, a slow realization or sudden illness. The implications were that the relationship assumed an inequality that was not previously present, the struggle to accept changes and a consequent immersion into the experience. Sonia says: *"I was running this now. I had to set the level of order, panic, urgency, control."*

Role Not Sought

Despite the need to be in control, one graphically sees that this is a role not sought, and this contributes to the way the accompanists accept the situation. Far from being easily accepted, it is one taken as a consequence of one's place within the relationship–the stronger person, the one who is not ill. Immersion means an all accepting taking on what *had* to be done; one reads of levels of panic rising and falling, and of unreal detachment, perhaps indicative of the shock of this life change. Ruth Cracknell describes: " . . . *my general feeling so detached, so unreal, so hazy–a complete sense of absence in other words–that . . . I felt like I might float off, up, to the ceiling . . . .* " Sonia experiences herself as "*a passenger there, for the ride, wherever it took me*" and contrary to her expectation of being able to rise to the challenges demanded of her, she is surprised that "*All the skills that had previously come so naturally to me had fallen away through unsteady grip; I had to re-teach myself the very basics. I had to show myself how to make pumpkin soup.*"

Letting Go

Immersion in a new role of caring meant basic changes in relationships and the loss of their old ways of being. Loss centred on what the relationship had been in the context of the accompanists life and the need to let it go. Sonia describes: *"I had let go, she had gone. I missed her, the old her. Missed talking to her, our laughter. But I didn't look for her anymore, expecting conversation, expecting anything."*

In the constant observation of the journey towards death, there endures the memory of what had gone before and an accompanying grief in this loss, especially the reciprocity of a more equal relationship. Kate says: "*I probably nursed the vain hope that he would become my partner again, rather than my charge, able to aid and comfort me as I him. Come back from wherever you're going, be adult and wise, understand how hard this is for me, too.*"

Loss was also characterised by unpredictability. For John, conversation required constant adaptation as Iris sank further into Alzheimer's. "*We can still talk as we did then, but it doesn't make sense any more, on either side. I can't reply in the way I used to, but only in the way she speaks to me now.*"

Unpredictability required flexibility and adaptation in the accompanying role, especially in relation to the progression of Alzheimer's disease. John continues: "*No sooner had we adjusted to life reduced in yet one more way than the wheel was spun again, to have another skill disappear, more memories eclipsed, setting in motion a new round of adapting.*"

Time is Meaningless

Time was vividly described in the stories as a characteristic of immersion, but a meaningless measurement that was happening for the caring person. Sonia says: "*I stumbled along–days? Weeks? A blur. I'm not sure. An amorphous existence where definition was lost, everything roughly edited, collaged onto one another. I was just existing, breathing in, out, in, out.*" Described as being in the midst of an uncertain, confused journey, Ruth says: "*I think we are, inescapably, on the last, unchartered journey–in the midst of it all when you really ache to halt time, time sometimes will be halted; but then you discover that it is not what you want either.*" The issue of time is particularly poignant for those with Alzheimer's, but felt not just by the person but also the carer, as John describes: "*When the Alzheimer's patient loses touch with time, time seems to lose both its prospective and its retrospective significance . . . for the partner that is.*"

The passing of time, too, is the constant reminder that it is running out, making each encounter precious. Ruth says: "*In those last days his desire to live every moment, to make it count, was inspiring and infectious.*" Ruth visits Eric in hospital, and observes: "*His eyes do not leave me and I begin to sing. . . . I go on and on waiting for the eyes to release me. For those hours . . . minutes–how many I have no idea of time, time had become meaningless."*

Immersion into the role is not accepted lightly, nor is it a constant, in the face of ever changing circumstances including the poignancy of the losses; it is where the accompanists' life is put on hold, in the face of the heavy demands of this role, which may go on and on.

Commitment–"A New Depth"

This theme describes the adaptation required from the accompanist in very basic aspects of their life and in ways that challenged and surprised them, even from within lengthy relationships.

Life Stripped Down

The emotional aspect of these changes makes particularly poignant reading, a sense of life being "stripped down" to its very basics. A keenly-felt loss of control is a frightening aspect of unfamiliar grief and each accompanist seemed to balance the need to be strong, with emotional "mess" at many levels. Ruth describes: *"Without warning I am filled with a sadness such as I have never known before, and sobs thrust from my gut–soundless, overwhelming."* And the pull between control and disintegration Sonia describes as: *"It felt good to cry. But the more I let myself relax deep into my sadness, the more I could feel my composure and strength inside. My emotional skeleton slowly disintegrated, I let myself fall."* And for Simone, the support from another was essential: *"I went home; talked to Sartre; we played some Bartok. Suddenly an outburst of tears that almost degenerated into hysteria."*

Life stripped down to essentials caused the accompanists to rail against separation from what had been the ordinariness of their life. The growing inability to enter into this ordinariness becomes a poignant reminder of what these carers have taken on separating them from life as it once was. Kate says: *"On the way home, I'd catch myself watching people hurrying along the street, preoccupied, places to go, mission to accomplish. Whatever their purpose, momentous or mundane, I envied them."* Simone describes the separation she felt from ordinary things: *"How desolate I was . . . in the cab that was taking me away! I knew this journey thru the fashionable quarters by heart. . . . Often the red light stopped me in front of Cardin's: I saw ridiculously elegant hats, waistcoats, scarves, slippers, shoes . . . jewels of a world in which death had no place; but it was there, lurking behind this façade, in the grey secrecy of the nursing homes, hospitals, sick rooms. And for me that was now the only truth."*

Within the stories chosen, fidelity within a partnered (marriage) relationship featured in three. This is not overtly spoken of however, rather it appears to be the strength drawn (perhaps *assumed*) from inside the relationship. John sees the irony of needing to work at the relationship, when he now has no choice. *"There is a certain comic irony–happily not darkly comic, that after 40 years of taking marriage for granted, marriage has decided it is tired of us and is taking a hand in the game. Purposely, persistently, involuntarily, our marriage is now getting somewhere. It is giving us no choice and I am glad of that."*

For Ruth, facing future battles together was a natural consequence of this commitment made a long time ago, and which added new depth. *". . . we had discovered a closeness–different–more intense than any experienced before, deeper even, than the height of our first passionate discoveries."*

Simplicity

In the relationship assuming a new depth, simplicity of action is required, often in the face of the constant suffering of this journey. Sonia, aware that death was near for Emma, *"went to bed . . . lay there, unable to sleep . . . wondering if I'd ever see her living again. I listened to her breath through the monitor. . . . Sometimes her breath was silent. . . . Then I'd hear a breath or two or very often a hiccup. And I'd smile. Emma is still here. I have her for one more day."*

After employing a carer, Kate says that: *"Now when I came to the home after work, instead of fussing with the hundred and one things his care entailed, I could sit quietly with him, watching the news or reading to him, usually poetry."*

The contained-ness of the partnership between carer and the cared for, is expressed in Ruth's words: *"In our isolated cocoon, he and I tunneled into one another. . . . There are times when we need nothing else."* And for Sonia the simple presence became a source of peace: *". . . I was enjoying her presence, simply that. I didn't need anything else. I knew I would value this moment later on. . . . The present moment consumed all my senses. . . . I didn't want it to end."*

Physical Proximity

Other times physical proximity was required to impart support. Aspects of physicality in the relationship appear to be part of the privilege and pain of being the accompanist: *"I climbed into bed with her, put my arm around her. I wished, wished so badly there was something, anything I could do,"* says Sonia. For Ruth, physical closeness to Eric was very important, and she describes how she achieved sleeping in the hospital with Eric and ensuring that their times apart were limited to as little as possible. *"There were nights when I would wake and realize that he was awake too. He never disturbed me and . . . I would try and soothe him to sleep."* And for Simone, the anguish of watching her mother's deteriorating body caused anxiety and discomfort that *"made her afraid of hurting her. . . . I took hold of that skeleton clothed under damp blue skin . . . standing on the side of the bed I held her and comforted her."*

But involvement in physical care called forth a surprising sensuality in its basic instinct to provide succor, as Ruth describes: *" I wrap gauze around my fingers, drench it in water and hold it to his lips . . . he sucks greedily and I repeat, repeat. . . . And from that moment the sucking has a satisfying pull on the teat, our tiny sensual moment."*

Silence

Silence had varying interpretations for the accompanists, for Sonia a symbol of a higher level of engagement with self: *"She was deep inside herself, departed from the outside world. And I watched, like a child, anxious for some attention. . . . The silence is a good sign, I kept reminding myself. She's dreaming, reinterpreting, meditating."*

Ruth's time with her children over lunch became a distraction and *"continued to soothe and strengthen. Sometimes we rarely spoke . . . we could even pretend we were on holiday–for a minute or two. . . . "* And Sonia's final acceptance that silence was an important part of Emma's journey to death: *"I didn't mind that we rarely spoke now. I was happy for her to be doing whatever it was that she needed to do."* The unspoken fusion of two people over a lifetime appears not to require words for Ruth: *"I am standing at the foot of his bed. I am alone with him. His eyes are open and he is holding my gaze with the greatest intensity I have experienced in our whole nearly forty-one years."*

New depths in an existing relationship appear to be a surprise for these accompanists, especially those with long and settled relationships. Life becomes reduced in its simplicity and expressions of presence become the most important priority.

Persistence–"Seeing Things Through"

The enduring nature of the caring relationship involves a constancy that creates overwhelming fatigue, a loss of confidence and challenges the accompanists' self-image. It means one's own desires and wishes become secondary to the tasks at hand.

Constancy

Constancy is graphically described by Sonia as holding oneself together: "*I was walking a tightrope with my past and future below me, balanced so precariously, sharpening my concentration, focusing on the job at hand.*" An aspect of constancy is overwhelming fatigue: "*I was so exhausted*" Ruth says " *. . . there's just no energy for anything else . . .*" Simone becomes ill and Kate remembers ". . . *how tired I was. I closed my eyes whenever I could. On the subway, in elevators, on escalators I slept like a horse, standing up.*"

Sonia's reaction to the constant caring is a loss of confidence: she considers that she has "*made a mistake. I shouldn't be here . . .*" and confusion at her inarticulation about what she wasn't coping with. "*The work didn't seem to stop. I have to ring Helen . . . to tell her to come and help me. Help me what: I don't know–just get me out of here. I was falling apart.*"

Of great difficulty to the accompanists was feeling an inadequate participant in the suffering, which called for a protective response. "*I'm so sick of this,*" Emma wept. "*I wasn't sure if she meant the illness, or the fight. Expectation, desire and hope were becoming luxuries for which we had less time or need. Once all else was removed, comfort and love were all I had. So with my arm around her, I wiped her face and wept with her–the only thing I had left to offer.*" Simone becomes "calmer" in the witness to her mother's suffering, once she knows what is happening "*The transition from my mother to a living corpse had definitely been accomplished. The world had shrunk to the size of her room . . . and it had only one aim–protecting her.*"

One's Own Needs on Hold

Persistence meant putting one's own needs put on hold, perhaps arising from a reciprocal sense–Sonia for example is aware of the small price she pays in putting her life on hold, given that–"*Em's been a great friend to me. . . . I'm sure she'd do the same.*" For Kate: "*My judgement was suspended, my tastes in literature, or anything else for that matter irrelevant. I didn't have the luxury.*" Simone's need to understand her mother's "*sickness and torment . . .* " cannot be met, because "*at the nursing home I did not have time to go into it. I had to help Maman to spit; I had to give her something to drink, arrange her pillows or her plat, move her leg, water her flowers, open the window, close it, read her the paper, answer her question, wind up her watch . . . but when I reached home all the sadness and horror of these last days dropped upon me with all its weight.*" Sonia's life change is expressed in: "*Remember when you could just sit with your friends and laugh about nothing?*" In presenting a brave face to the world she is "*torn, juggling, hiding a mind in crisis behind a screened face. People say I am strong. I am not strong. I am crumbling.*"

Self Image

The accompanist's self image is challenged and changed by the caring role, expressed in the fluctuating levels of confidence felt in being faithful to the ill person, confronted with the stark reality of what they had taken on. "*I didn't know how to do this*" says Sonia. "*I'm the wrong person for the job; I came here to be with Emma–not for this. She was not her old self and I was a stranger. I am her carer.*"

The changes that taking on this caring role had wrought are described in terms of personal growth. Kate makes a self-observation that: "*Alzheimer's was surely sent to teach me patience, not one of my virtues. I was getting good at it though, not even feeling irritation. . . .* " Sonia says: "*I am a different person. . . . I have been forced to go somewhere new inside–an increased level of sadness has etched itself into me–right to the very edges. . . . I no longer feel that my life is destined for any kind of greatness. But I feel more human than ever before.*"

One gets a glimpse of healing for Simone when she describes that she "*had grown fond of this dying woman. As we talked in the half-darkness I assuaged an old unhappiness; I was renewing the dialogue that had been broken off during my adolescence and that our differences and our likenesses had never allowed us to take up again.*"

These three themes describe aspects of intimate fidelity within the caring role, when taken on in a one-to-one relationship. Although these themes find little echo in the academic and professional literature, the stories chosen have provided ample material rich in experience, for thematic analysis. In writing about their caring roles, intimate carers offer their reflective experience, from which others in such roles may learn.

PROFESSIONAL FIDELITY

Although specialist nursing roles exist where nurses use all their professional time to care for dying people, the concept of fidelity is not used in descriptions of these roles. Using the literature on professional caring, commonalities and differences in intimate fidelity and professional fidelity are highlighted, using the themes developed.

Immersion

While professional carers would not usually describe their caring roles as being so consuming that life is "put on hold," one could argue that the concept of being immersed in a professional caring role is never-the-less valid in other ways. Benner and Wrubel's work (1989) on caring describes qualities of knowing the patient, being with another in an engaged manner, doing for them what they cannot so for themselves and enabling what needs to be done for their own health. These aspects of care may be understood as essential interpretations of being immersed into the ill person's experience.

Chapman's work (1998) on palliative care nurses describes "presencing" as an important aspect of "being there" referring to the nature of the time spent, as being more than the physical presence, extending to being able to identify with and understand the experience of the ill person. Presencing involves being flexible in response to individual situations; thus, patterns of responses become less useful. Again, drawing on the thematic analysis, the immersion required of presencing may be a simple gesture, such as sitting with the person.

Chapman (1998) also describes the attitude of open questioning–of one's own experiences and oneself–as the basis of acceptance adaptability. Additionally, acceptance and non-judgmental attitudes assist nurses in immersing themselves into the individual person's experience to facilitate their choices and care.

Commitment

Palliative care literature describes the development of "modern palliative care" (somewhere during the mid-late 1970s) as providing an opportunity for individuals to respond to the challenge, seen at the time as akin to a human rights movement, to improve care for dying people (O'Connor, 2001). Vachon (1995) notes that many of these people were fired with a desire, akin to a "calling," because of a personal experience, to work with a charismatic leader, or because of particular values systems, translated into an enduring commitment. These staff reported great satisfaction in being able to impact on an individual's quality of life, and assisting them to come to terms with their impending death. These kinds of satisfactions are reported as the rewards of working in palliative care and find echoes in the commitment aspect of the role of intimate fidelity.

Persistence

While there is a different emphasis on the characteristic of persistence found in the professional literature, resonances with descriptions in intimate caring roles are also found. The constancy of professional fidelity in caring roles exhibits itself as a stressor, and the literature contains significant work on coping with caring roles (Vachon, 1995; Chapman, 1998; O'Connor & Aranda, 2003). There are clear directions in the literature about ways to assist palliative care professionals to cope with their roles (Aranda, 2000; Lee, 1998; Vachon, 2001). Korbasa (1979) describes the characteristic of "hardiness" as central to one's ability to cope with continually difficult work–characterised by commitment, control, and challenge. Adequate educational preparation for dealing with issues of dying and grief is of prime importance (Power & Sharp, 1988), using reflective learning styles, incorporating problem-based learning principles, and models that utilise those people with advanced practice skills (Lee, 1998).

The development of effective teamwork is seen as a major difference in intimate and professional caring roles: the stories of intimate caring highlighting the isolation and aloneness of their role, whereas team support is central in professional roles. This involves a time commitment to the development of effective interactions between team members and agreed rules and working conditions, a commitment to make them work, and recognition from management. One aspect of a team's agenda ought to be about how they will provide collegial support to each other: different in each team, but overt, understood and agreed by each team member. This is an expression of collegial fidelity that is worthy of further reflection in relation to the needs of intimate carers.

The aspect of the balance of one's own life has received some attention in the literature (Vachon, 1995). In recognising the sometimes burdensome aspects of care, individuals need to take responsibility for creating balance–be it in life-giving hobbies and regular exercise, working part-time, taking regular time-out, and being disciplined in undertaking regular self-reflection. This is a serious responsibility, which no one else can do for the individual, but professional colleagues can gently lead by example and sharing the wisdom of their experience. The ability to learn from others in professional environments is quite different from the experience of intimate carers; from the writings utilised in this article, the caring experience seems to be dominated by isolation, loneliness and being overwhelmed by what they had taken on.

While professional fidelity finds some commonality with intimate fidelity, some differences are also obvious. The most important is that of the supports that are assumed as part of professional caring roles–informal collegiality and shared work structures like teams and formalized educational programs. This is an important consideration when thinking about support of intimate caring roles in moving into the future where intimate caring roles may well become more common as community caring roles become more a part of the community fabric.

COMMUNAL FIDELITY: CARING FOR OUR MOST VULNERABLE

Communal fidelity is the level in the model that encompasses policy and institutional manifestations of fidelity. It is often anecdotally suggested that a community is judged by the way it cares for its most vulnerable. Like many hidden aspects of community structures, faithful caring is mostly unacknowledged and unrewarded if undertaken in an un-contentious manner. If caring is not according to communal expectations however, or is found wanting, then media headlines decry the carers or their organisations and the community is outraged. For example, a nursing home was closed as a result of a media campaign which revealed that a resident's scabies had been treated by immersion in a kerosene bath (Hodge, 2000). Communal fidelity encompasses the systems and processes that enable carers–both intimate and professional–to undertake their roles. Unless seen in policies that enable carers to undertake their tasks, communal fidelity may remain unspoken (Heaton, 1999).

Heaton (1999) notes that over recent years there has been a notable shift in the locus of care, from the institution to the community, with growing communal supports aimed to keep people in their own homes for longer periods. This is noted as a philosophical change from "care *in* the community to care *by* the community" (p. 761) and the consequent development of informal (intimate) caring roles, including incorporation of such roles in government policies. Policy has differentiated between formal (or professional) carers and informal carers, the latter being viewed as "unpaid carers who provide care out of love and filial piety" (Harrington, 1999, 765). However, recent policy has incorporated the needs of informal carers as users of services too.

McNamara (2001) and O'Connor (2004) note the different communal emphases between the way younger dying and older dying are provided with care. For younger dying people efforts are made to provide all aspects of holistic care required by them and their families, being regarded as an "undeserved death." For older people, the death is expected, seen to be the end of a life lived, and thus at some level, requiring less of our expertise–"the decrepit death" (O'Connor, 2004).

In relation to the concept of commitment, of note in the palliative care literature is the historical view of the early days of care of the dying in Australia–care of the dying was mostly provided by the religious orders from the earliest days of health care, simply because it was not regarded as a priority–it was work that interested no one else (Smith, 2000). The work remained passive comfort care, hidden and mostly unacknowledged in large hospices in most capital cities. In its own way though, early care of the dying in Australia was a testimony of un-trumpeted fidelity to those forgotten at the end of life.

In relation to intimate carers, a visible example of policy support in 2004 is the over $2m that has been allocated over the 5 years of the current Australian Health Care Agreement (2003-8) for initiatives in palliative care, including increasing resources for respite. The increase in the carers pension in the 2004 Federal Budget (while many would argue is still inadequate), is another commitment to the often taken-for-granted contribution of intimate carers to the community.

Palliative Care Australia recently released a study into the "Social Impact of Caring for Terminally Ill People in Australia" (2004) and noted that carers contribute over $20 billion to the Australian economy. The study found many hidden costs, financial, social and emotional. "Carers' health and wellbeing seems inextricably linked to the availability, quality, responsiveness and cost of support from health and community services" (p. 9). The study made several policy recommendations, including:

- Policy developments in areas like taxation, social security, workplace and income/pension benefit domains;
- Coordination of funding and service provision across levels of government, to link policy and practice and to develop standards for service quality;

- Education strategies for carers and for health professionals (p. 7).

Another important communal expression of commitment to those at the end of life is that of spiritual and religious support provided. McNamara (2001) notes that spiritual needs of people facing the end of life are the least understood, mainly because " in our increasing secular society dying and death are relegated by the state and sub-sumed within scientific discourses" (p. 59). In keeping with the holistic philosophy of palliative care, spiritual suffering is as important as physical pain; thus, pastoral care roles ought to be very visible in specialist palliative care teams. Some particular faith traditions that utilize rituals to mark key life passages, however, are finding that often because of person-power issues, they cannot honour end of life rituals, so often considered an essential support in dying, especially by older people. This sinister and unjust tragedy needs serious examination by faith institutions and new models of ritualistic support are urgently required.

Thus there is a *growing* recognition of the necessity for developing community structures that will support and recognise individuals within the community who are caring for people in both intimate and professional roles; however, there is certainly much more work to be achieved.

CONCLUSION

The use of narrative has been an eclectic way to begin to describe the concept of fidelity, particularly at the level of intimate fidelity. Aspects of this concept are not readily found in professional literature. Perhaps this oversight is indicative of how much we take fidelity for granted–at intimate, professional and communal levels? Even though there are hopeful signs, there is much work to be undertaken that will provide consistent linkages between the layers of intimate, professional, and communal fidelity. In honouring the hidden sacrifice so inherent in faithful, intimate caring, this is an area where creative research could complement the concept that has been proposed here.

Characteristics of fidelity–immersion, commitment, and persistence–remind us of the suffering and difficulties and rewards which come with accompanying a person on the journey to death.

REFERENCES

Aranda, S. (2000). Palliative nursing in Australia. In: A. Kellehear (Ed.), *Death & dying in Australia*. Melbourne: Oxford University Press.

Bayley, J. (1998). *Iris: A memoir of Iris Murdoch*. London: Abacus books.

Beauchamp, T., & Childress, J. (1989). *Principles of biomedical ethics (3rd ed.). New York: Oxford University Press.*

Benner, P., & Wrubel, J. (1989). *The primacy of caring*. California: Addison-Wesley.

Borkan, J., Reis, S., Steinmetz, D., & Medalie, J. (1999). *Patients and doctors: Life changing stories from primary care*. Wisconsin: University of Wisconsin Press.

Brewer, E. C. (1898). The Fidelity mantle. In: *Dictionary of phrase and fable*. Philadelphia: Henry Altemus Company.

Chapman, Y. (1998). Nursing dying people. In: J. Parker & S. Aranda (Eds.), *Palliative care: Explorations and challenges*. Sydney: McLennan and Petty.

Cracknell, R. (2000). *Journey from Venice: A memoir*. Melbourne: Penguin Books.

De Beauvoir, S. (1964). *A very easy death*. London: Penguin Books.

Delbridge, A. (Ed.). (1986). *The Macquarie dictionary*. New South Wales: Macquarie University.

Franks, A. (1995) *The wounded storyteller: Body illness & ethics*. Chicago: University of Chicago Press.

Heaton, J. (1999). The gaze and visibility of the carer: A Foucauldian analysis of the discourse of informal care. *Sociology of Health and Illness, 21/6*, 759-777.

Hodge, A. (8th March 2000). Nurses burned by kerosene episode: The nursing home scandal. *The Australian*, p. 4.

Jennings, K. (2003). *Moral hazard*. Sydney: Picador.

Kearney, R. (2002). *On stories*. London: Routledge.

Korbasa, S. C. (1979). Stressful life events, personality, and health: An inquiry into hardiness. *Journal of Personality & Social Psychology, 37*, 1-11 National Hospice.

Lee, S. (1998). Expertise in palliative care nursing: A nursing view of the generalist/specialist debate. In: J. Parker & S. Aranda (Eds.), *Palliative care: Explorations and challenges*. Sydney: McLennan & Petty.

McNamara, B. (2001). *Fragile lives: Death, dying, and care*. Sydney: Allen & Unwin.

O'Connor, M., & Aranda, S. (2003). *Palliative care nursing: A guide to practice*. Melbourne: Ausmed Publications.

O'Connor, M. (2001). *The veils of death: Understanding dying in residential aged care–A discourse analysis of policy*. Unpublished thesis, Melbourne: La Trobe University.

O'Connor, M. (2004). Ageing in place, dying in place: The clash of philosophy and practice in aged and palliative care. In: S. Nelson (Ed.), *Ethics, power, practice: In sickness and in health series*. Bournemouth: Nursing Praxis International.

Orchard, S. (2003). *Something more wonderful: A true story*. Sydney: Hodder.

Palliative Care Australia (2004). *The hardest thing I have ever done: The social impact of caring for terminally ill people in Australia*. Canberra: Palliative Care Australia.

Pellegrino, E., & Thomasma, D. (1993). *The virtues of medical practice*. New York: Oxford University Press.

Power, K. G., & Sharp, G. R. (1988). A comparison of sources of nursing stress and job satisfaction among mental handicap and hospice nursing staff. *Journal of Advanced Nursing, 13*, 726-32.

Ramsey, P. (1970). *The patient as person.* New Haven: Yale University Press.

Smith, D. (2001). *Once in each lifetime.* Melbourne: MEPCA.

Smith, M. (2000). Death, health policy, and palliative care. In: A. Kellehear (Ed.), *Death & dying in Australia.* Melbourne: Oxford University Press.

Vachon, M. L. S. (1995). Staff stress in hospice/palliative care. *Palliative Medicine, 9,* 91-122.

Vachon, M. L. S. (2001). The world of palliative care nursing. In: B. Rolling-Ferrell, & N. Coyle (Eds.), *Textbook of palliative care nursing.* New York: Oxford University Press.

Index

Accountability, 209
Activities, continuity of, 22,25
Adaptation, to aging, 25-26
Afterlife, belief in
    death anxiety and, 98,103-104
    religiousness and, 100,102,103
    spirituality and, 102
Agape, 41,157,181-182
Ageism, 33
Aggression, dementia-related, 81
Aging
    adaptation to, 25-26
    depressive perspective on, 13-14
    individual perspective on, 12
    life-cycle model of, 35
    negative perceptions of, 10-12
    positive perceptions of, 12-13
    problem-based theory of, 10-12
    schematic social history of, 34-36
    successful/positive, 11,33,35,97
    tasks and purpose of, 14,67-68
Alzheimer's patients
    caregivers' fidelity toward, 231,
        233,234,235,237-238
    palliative care for, 191
    perception of time by, 76
    personal accounts of, 74-75
American Indians, 112
Anglican Retirement Community
    Services, 80
An Imaginary Life (Malouf), 55
Anomie, 11-12
Antonovsky, A., 14
Aristotle, 160
Art, spiritual and healing properties of,
    28,67-68
Arthur, King of Britain, 229
Art of Play, The (Blatner and Blatner),
    150-151

Australia, end-of-life palliative care in
    Australian Health Care Agreement
        and, 242
    Australian Palliative Residential
        Aged Care (APRAC) Project,
        191-192,201,202-203
    caregivers in, 242-243
    Clown Doctors program in,
        137-152
    for dementia patients, 194-195
    historical background to, 242
    National Health and Medical
        Research Council and, 197
    Palliative Care Australia, 242-243
    spiritual care in, 61-62
Australian Health Care Agreement,
    242
Australian Palliative Residential Aged
    Care (APRAC) Project,
    191-192,201,202-203

Baby-boomer generation, 132
Barth, Karl, 48
Beauvoir, de, Simone,
    231,234-235,236,238
Belief in Afterlife scale, 99
Belief systems, effect of life-limiting
    illness on, 131
Bereavement support, 198-200
    for dementia patients, 199
Bible, 164-165
    New Testament, 160,164
    Old Testament, 164
Bio-ethics, concept of fidelity in, 230
Biomedical model, of health care,
    119-121
Bird Dementia Scale, 83

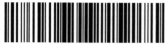

Made in the USA
Middletown, DE
14 November 2018